Cooperation versus rivalry in times of pandemic

Edited by

Radosław Fiedler
Sang Chul Park
Artur Pohl

Logos Verlag Berlin

λογος

Reviewer
Prof. Arkadiusz Żukowski

Coordinators of the publishing project
Artur Pohl
Radosław Fiedler

English language consultancy
Roma K. Kwiatkiewicz
Catharine Haitzmann

Bibliographic information published by Die Deutsche Bibliothek

Bibliografische Information der Deutschen Nationalbibliothek
Die Deutsche Nationalbibliothek verzeichnet diese Publikation
in der Deutschen Nationalbibliografie; detaillierte bibliografische Daten
sind im Internet über http://dnb.d-nb.de abrufbar.

The research was financed from the project „Research on COVID-19" from the funds
of the Adam Mickiewicz University, Poznań

ISBN 978-3-8325-5291-6

Logos Verlag Berlin GmbH
Georg-Knorr-Str. 4, Geb. 10
D-12681 Berlin
Germany

Tel.: +49 (0) 30/42 85 10 90
Fax: +49 (0) 30/42 85 10 92

http://www.logos-verlag.com

CONTENTS

Sang-Chul Park
Korea Polytechnic University

COOPERATION VERSUS COMPETITION: PRECONDITIONS FOR BALANCED GLOBAL POLITICS[1]

Politics are regarded as a comprehensive art orchestrated by various actors such as leading, supporting, participating roles, etc. It is also a state of art how to compromise, protect and arrange national interests among and between nations. Therefore, it is very significant to understand how world politics are structured and operated in order to protect and maximize their interests as well as maintain peace and the status quo. Since the Second World War, the new world order was created by the U.S. leadership based on her overwhelming economic and military dominance that lasted till the end of the twentieth century. However, the global political situation started to change dramatically with the end of the Cold War caused by the collapse of the Berlin Wall in 1989.

After the harsh competition between the East and the West, the U.S. established unilateral world leadership, although the European Union (EU) attempted to create the political union of United Europe at the beginning of the 2000s to challenge the U.S. leadership in global politics. Unfortunately, the EU's political union could not be realized once France and the Netherlands rejected it. At the same time, however, the EU has remained the largest economic bloc and had competed with the U.S. in terms of the global economy, until Brexit was realized in 2016. Despite its economic primacy before and the current position of being the second-largest economy in terms of size, the EU has a fundamental weakness because it does not have any

---

[1] The research was financed from the project „Research on COVID-19" from the funds of the Adam Mickiewicz University, Poznan

unified financial system at the EU level. Under such circumstances, China emerged as the second-largest economy in 2010.

Since then, the U.S. has been facing challenges to the economic superpower due to the rise of China. After China started its open policy in 1978, China's economic scale, foreign trade, and technological development have been growing rapidly. As a result, it took over German position as the third-largest economy in 2009 and a year later became the second largest in the world, which was rather dramatic and very fast. China's role in the global economy has grown to be even more significant particularly since the global financial crisis (GFC) in 2008 because the major economies such as the U.S., the EU, Japan, Korea suffered from the long term sluggish economic conditions after the GFC. Compared to the low economic low growth in the advanced countries, China generated high and medium levels of economic growth till the mid of the 2010s. Therefore, it is widely recognized that the bilateral relationship between the USA and China will be a crucial determinant of the world's direction in the twenty-first century because China has tried to build a new form of the cooperative platform in world politics and the global economy by creating G2 in 2013 when President Xi, Jinping took the power. (Kirton, 2013; Xi, 2017; Park, 2020, 2021).

Under the Obama government, G2 Summit was held regularly, and China pushed hard to be recognized as a competitor and a partner to the U.S. The EU's position on how to deal with such a structural transformation in the world was unclear because the EU had to tackle its own agenda to solve economic difficulties after the GFC and the sovereign debt crisis in 2010/2011. Under such a power vacuum, China moved fast to strengthen its economic and political leadership in East Asia by negotiating the trilateral FTA between China, Japan, and Korea as well as the Mega FTA of RCEP, in order to compete with the U.S.-led TPP in Asia and create a regional economic integration led by China. At the same time, China initiated the One Belt and One Road Project (OBOR) in 2013 that turned to the Belt and Road Initiative (BRI) in 2018. The BRI is an ambitious project connecting over 100 countries by six land and three sea routes and represents the Chinese dream as an economic and political superpower along with the USA in the twenty-first century. For it, President Xi addressed in the Summit with President Obama in Washington D. C. in 2013 that the Pacific is big and wide enough to share for two superpowers with each other. Unfortunately, however, President Obama did not understand what it means. Since then, China has tried hard to realize its dream coming true and expand its military bases in the

Southeast Sea or South China Sea that was claimed strongly by Southeast Asian neighbor countries as well as other major powers such as the USA, the EU, Japan, and Australia. (Asia Development Bank, 2017; OECD, 2018; Chinese Government, 2016; Xi, 2017; Zong, 2020).

To become a real superpower, China needed to develop and upgrade the industry because its industrial structure was still weak in terms of high-tech areas. Still, China has to import approximately 70% of high-tech parts and components in order to complete its end products to export to the advanced markets. China imports these mainly from Korea, Japan, Taiwan, the U.S., and the EU. Such a structural weakness was regarded as Achilles Hill for Chinese further development. Therefore, China set up its industrial long-term plan known as China Manufacturing 2025 focusing on strategic high tech areas such as 5G telecommunication technology, AI, IoT, big data, advanced robotics, etc. that are closely related to the Fourth Industrial Revolution (FIR).

In order to catch up with the technological level of advanced countries, China tried to purchase foreign companies through aggressive M & A, as well as strongly demanded that foreign companies operating in China transfer high technologies, treating them in a discriminative manner and generally – unfairly, compared with the treatment of domestic companies in China. The Chinese government has provided financial subsidies only to Chinese companies and excluded foreign companies operating in China to catch up with the technological level of advanced countries. Given the rule of WTO, it violates the Most Favored Nation Clause. Therefore, developed countries started to suspect Chinese M & A approaches in the high technology sectors and felt threatened on the level of national security. Finally, they suspended Chinese purchases in national security-related industries. Since then, trade conflicts and disputes between China and advanced countries have rapidly increased.

The Trump Administration started the trade war with China by exposing high tariffs to Chinese imports and vice versa in 2017, which lasted till the end of his government in January of 2021. The new Biden government expressed clearly that the U.S. trade policy is based on the Buy American Products instead of America First carried out by the Trump Administration. It means that the Biden government is ready to fight against Chinese unfair trade behaviors violating the U.S. IPRs and discriminating against the U.S. companies' business activities in China. It means that the trade conflicts between the two economic superpowers will continue in the near future as long as the U.S. maintains its hardline approach towards China in terms of the trade policy. Logically, it is foreseeable that the Biden government will continue to protect the U.S. strategic high-tech industries in order to prevent China from accessing these areas.

Ever since 2020, and under these circumstances, the world has been experiencing the COVID-19 pandemic, which has negatively affected the global economy on a scale that hadn't been experienced ever since the Great Depression in 1929. The Chinese lockdown in early 2020 resulted in severe damage to global value chains (GVCs) and regional value chains (RVCs) because China has played as the global factory for the world economy since the 2000s. As a result, advanced countries started to rethink how to restore and rebuild the GVCs and the RVCs excluding China. The COVID-19 pandemic will harm the global economy in various ways. First of all, the rearrangement of GVCs and RVCs will increase additional production costs for producers, which would reduce the consumption power and economic growth in the long run. Secondly, the pandemic could cause high asset inflation because most countries have expanded their monetary and financial policy measures to maintain their sluggish economies. However, to a high extent, the capital has not been allocated in the production side, but either in the stock market or the property market. Last, but not least the pandemic accelerated the Fourth Industrial Revolution (FIR) using ICT technologies more than ever to create hyper automation and hyper-connectivity that enabled the creation of the digital economy across the world much faster than expected. (Park, 2018; 2021).

To realize the FIR, all nations need to purchase semiconductor products that are the core and key products to all high-tech areas. Therefore, these are regarded as oil in the 21st century. Korea supplied highly sophisticated semiconductor products around 22 percent of the global supply, while Taiwan with 21% and the U.S. with 12% in 2020. In total, Korea and Taiwan supplied around 43% of highly sophisticated semiconductor products globally and became the hub of the semiconductor industry. Therefore, the U.S. and China are both trying to convince Korea to become their major economic partner supplying the key products stable in the long run. For Korea, China is the largest export market, ahead of the U.S. and the EU on a global scale, the market which generates the largest share of trade surplus among its trade partners. However, Korea does not share its national interest in terms of politics based on democracy and human rights as well as security based on the military support with China. On the contrary, the U.S. is Korea's most important strategic ally for its national security and political system as well as its second-largest trade partner. It means that China is important for Korea only in its national economy, while the U.S. for economic, military, and political interests.

Therefore, Korea has to keep the balance between the two superpowers in order to maximize its national interests, which is possible as long as Korea maintains its position in developing key products based on high-technology development continuously. The best scenario for Korea is that the two superpowers will find a status quo or peaceful cooperation and economically competitive relationship for the global economy. In fact, it is the precondition for stable global politics and economy for all nations. Unfortunately, however, the best scenario seems to be not taken into account at present, due to the harsh competition of economic and political hegemony between the two superpowers starting from the trade conflicts, through the financial conflict, and possibly going all the way to a military conflict. Therefore, this situation is rather a long-term one. In this case, the second-best scenario, which is to keep the balance between the superpowers, seems to be more realistic in the near future. It means that Korea faces a challenge in how to keep its technological and production leadership, in the context of supplying key products, which the two economic superpowers will absolutely need to purchase for their national interest in the future, on a continuous basis.

References

Asia Development Bank (ADB) (2017), *Meeting Asia's Infrastructure Needs*, www.adb.org/sites/default/files/publication/227496/special-report-infrastructure.pdf., (accessed on 06 March 2021).

Chinese Government (2016), *China's National Plan on Implementation of the 2030 Agenda for Sustainable Development*, www.fmprc.gov.cn/web/ziliao_674904/zt_674979/dnzt_674981/qtzt/2030kcxfzyc_686343/P02017041468 9023442403.pdf., (accessed on 08 March 2021).

Kirton J. (2013), *G20 Governance for a Globalized World*, Farnham: Ashgate.

OECD (2018) *China's Belt and Road Initiative in the Global Trade, Investment and Finance Landscape*, OECD Business and Finance Outlook 2018, Paris.

Park S-C (2018), *The Fourth Industrial Revolution and Implications for Innovative Cluster Policies*, "AI & Society", Vol. 33, No. 3, pp. 433–445

Park S-C (2020), *Trade Conflict Between the U.S. and China: What are the Impacts on the Chinese Economy? International Organizations Research Journal*, Vol. 15, No. 2, pp. 153–168

Park S-C (2021), *Asian Regional Cooperation: RCEP and CPTPP Strategy after Brexit*, in: Haba K. and Holland M. (eds.) *Brexit and After: Perspectives on European Crises and Reconstruction from Asia and Europe*, Singapore: Springer.

Xi J. P. (2017), *Secure a Decisive Victory in Building a Moderately Prosperous Society in all Respects and Strive for the Great Success of Socialism with Chinese Characteristics for a New Era*, Delivered at the 19th National Congress of the Communist Party of China, 18 October,

Zhong Y. (2020), *The European Union and the South China Sea Dispute: A Case for Balancing with European Characteristics*, "Asia Pacific Journal of EU Studies", Vol. 18, No. 3.

Radosław Fiedler
Adam Mickiewicz University, Poznan
ORCID 0000-0003-1573-9898

COMPETITION OR COOPERATION IN THE COVID-19 (POST)-PANDEMIC WORLD[1]

The world in November 2019 was in a satisfying economic shape, although this does not mean that there were no threats to undermine this global economic growth. The annual growth of the global economy was almost 3% (International Monetary Fund 2019). Moreover, the total international tourist arrivals reached 1,4 billion in 2019 (International tourism receipts, plus passenger transport) altogether of an extremely high amount of USD 1.7 trillion (International Tourism Highlights 2019). Another example of very intensive connectivity was the busiest air traffic on July 25, 2019, with more than 230, 000 flights taken around the globe. It was the busiest day in the history of aviation. Almost 90% of goods in global trade are carried by the ocean shipping industry each year. Just in November 2019, before the COVID-19 pandemic, we enjoyed the benefits of intensification of connections, mass tourism, the business that knows no borders, free movement of capital, people, services, and technology, have argued that the world has not only got smaller but is also intertwined in many different ways and that the process of globalization cannot be reversed. Indicators showing the multidimensionality of globalization is much more, such as capital flows, international trade, offshoring, globalization of production, and the most important message of the whole process has to be primarily beneficial to the key actors which are transnational corporations (Fiedler 2020: 5).

Globalization as a multidimensional process has been accelerated by big corporations due to the apparent economic and financial apparent advan-

---

[1] The research was financed from the project „Research on COVID-19" from the funds of the Adam Mickiewicz University, Poznan

tages. As noted by Robert Reich, American corporations have no special allegiance to the United States and no responsibility for the well-being of Americans, but having an impact on US politics (Reich 2020: 61). As he accounted, American-based global corporations added 2.4 million workers outside the United States in the first decade of the twenty-first century while cutting their American workforce by 2.9 million. Nearly 60% of their revenue growth has come from outside of America. Apple employs 43,000 people in the United States but has more than 700,000 workers contracted abroad (Reich 2020: 61–63). The main concern now is to indicate the taxation of corporation and closure of the possibilities of registering income in tax havens.

What should be especially emphasized from January 2020, is that the rise of the COVID-19 pandemic forced the closure of factories, warehouses, ports, airports, and many different sectors, which has resulted in enormous disruptions in global supply chains. It is still very difficult to assess all the effects of COVID-19, as the pandemic is an ongoing global challenge, and reprocessing of enormous data is needed. Also, we deal with many variables and their negative impact on the life of individuals and society. Social groups need to be analyzed, and a separate issue would be data collection on children and adolescents, specifically their disrupted relationships due to social distancing, and the effects of online education. Are we dealing with a generation that is less successful in social, personal, and professional life? Besides, many industries have suffered and still are suffering severe losses and it is not clear yet in what condition and whether they will return to economic activity. This concerns primarily the tourism, culture, and gastronomy industries. The civil airline industry is an illustration of a deep crisis. In 2019, it had a capacity for 4.5 billion passengers and over 100,000 air connections a day – globally, the industry employed 10 million people, not including additional services as follows: TAXI, gastronomy, multiple information and logistics services, and many others offering services and subcontractors of giant airport terminals - generating approximately income of $ 170 billion (Economist, August 1, 2020).

Due to economic forecasts, the coronavirus crisis will leave emerging economies on average 4 % smaller in 2024 than has been expected before the pandemic. Losses in Latin America will be over 6% and almost 8% in emerging Asia with the exception of China (Gliles 2021). The post-pandemic world could face renewed social tensions and rising instability both on an internal and regional level.

In this context, the COVID-19 crisis was specified as a "reallocation shock" due to the decision to freeze all sectors of economic and professional activity requiring personal contacts, such as e.g. tourism, airlines, hotel industry, gastronomy, entertainment, and culture industry. They have been subjected to a specific and long-term shock and it would be very difficult to revert to pre-pandemic indicators (Barrero, Bloom, Davis 2020). Another problem that the COVID-19 pandemic has recalled is strained supply chains and the additionally deepening rivalry between the US and China. For example, maritime transport, which is crucial for international trade, and above all the growing demand for container ships, increased the costs of container transport by over 100% (Stephens 2021). While disruptions in supply chains had occurred before, they were short-lived and more local and related to natural disasters. For example, the IT industry and the temporary disruptions in the supply of hard drives, due to the flooding in Thailand, and the Fukushima earthquake was affected by disruptions in the supply of electronics and chemicals.

Almost global lockdown introduced between March and April 2020 and the shock it had in global supply chains, as well as competition for limited and strategic reserves of medical and protective equipment, has sparked in-depth reflection on whether the current model of globalization and excessive dispersion of suppliers is not a threat for the security of supply? Could globalization transform into a more oriented regional supply chain? How to define the strained relations additionally fueled by the strategic US-China rivalry?

The COVID-19 pandemic should enable more cooperative international relations. Unfortunately, on the one hand, the tensions have increased, on the other, cooperation is essential for global vaccination programs, for economic recovery, and a more stable and predictable international system. The state actors like China and the US tend to forget that without strong cooperation, it may be difficult to regain the positive economic indicators from 2019. Before the pandemic, climate change represented an existential threat for which global leadership is unprepared. The pandemic has revealed multiple failures in the national and global response to the COVID-19 pandemic. Moreover, Erik Nielsen, the chief economist of UniCredit, drew attention to the issue of the virus and its possible new variants which would put a risk for the fragile recovery. In his opinion, the global economy remains a highly uncertain and risky place as it emerges from the pandemic (Gliles 2021).

Needless to say, one of the most positive and apparent effects of the pandemic and the enforced lockdowns is the fact that even though digitization processes, the development of artificial intelligence (AI), automation and robotization, and remote work technologies had already taken place before the COVID-19, and the pandemic accelerated and deepened these trends and probably significantly shorten the period needed for that to happen. Indeed, progress that has come about within a year of the pandemic, would probably take five years under normal circumstances (Nübler, 2020: 192).

Analyzing the different trends of the world during and after a pandemic should not be an unnecessary intellectual exercise. For this purpose, within an interdisciplinary and international team, we have undertaken a study of the project: "Research on COVID-19" conducted at Adam Mickiewicz University, Poznan in Poland.

Therefore, the scientific objectives of the project include:

1. Determining the nature and scale of the impact of the pandemic on the international order, with particular emphasis on the patterns of cooperation and competition between its actors.
2. Analysis of multi-level decisions in response to a pandemic crisis.
3. Identification of the effects of health policies and the changes they cause on the functioning of societies in the context of international interactions.

This publication is the result of the work of the research team that undertook the task of analyzing the COVID-19 pandemic effects from various perspectives: national, regional, and global. The analysis also should contribute to a better understanding of the nature of post-pandemic international relations and as a guideline for different stakeholders: decision-makers from local and state level, journalists, scholars, students, and all of the readers who would like to educate and be active in their communities.

References

Air travel's sudden collapse will reshape a trillion-dollar industry (2020), https://www.economist.com/business/2020/08/01/air-travels-sudden-collapse-will-reshape-a-trillion-dollar-industry, (accessed March 10, 2021).

Balzhan S., Kanat A., Yessengali O. (2020), *State Capacity in Responding to COVID-19*, "International Journal of Public Administration".

Barrero J., Bloom M, Davis S. (2020), *COVID-19 Is Also a Reallocation Shock, Brookings Papers on Economic Activity*, Summer 2020.

Bigger than Trump. The White House v covid-19Now that the Trump administration has taken charge of the government's pandemic response, how is it doing? (2020), https://www.economist.com/united-states/2020/04/11/the-white-house-v-covid-19, (accessed March 10, 2021).

Beck U. (2000), *What is globalization?* Cambridge, UK, Malden, MA: Polity Press. Blyth, Mark, 2020.

Cohen S. (2021), *Looking Back and Looking Ahead After a Year of Pandemic* https://blogs.ei.columbia.edu/2021/03/08/looking-back-looking-ahead-year-pandemic, (accessed March 10, 2021).

Fiedler R. (2020), *From corportationism to cooperationism: reversed globalization, cooperative politics and expanding online communication in post-pandemic time*, "Society Register", 4 (3).

Giles Ch. (2021), *This crisis is different: the dramatic rebound in the global economy*, "Financial Times", https://www.ft.com/content/f99210c9-c909–4325–8f6b-6684faabef0a, (accessed April 10, 2021).

International Tourism Highlights (2019), https://www.e-unwto.org/doi/pdf/10.18111/9789284421152, (accessed March 10, 2021).

Nübler I. (2020), *Shaping the Work of the Future: Policy Implications*, (in:) *Work in the Future The Automation Revolution*, ed. Robert Skidelsky and Nan Craig, Palgrave Macmillan.

Reich R. (2020), *The System. Who Rigged It, How We Fix It*, Alfred A. Knopf, New York.

Why America's Growth Model Suggests It Has Few Good Options (2020) "Foreign Policy", March 30, https://www.foreignaffairs. com/articles/americas/2020–03–30/us-economy-uniquely, (accessed March 10, 2021).

Sang-Chul Park
Korea Polytechnic University
ORCID: 0000-0002-4572-9036

THE TRADE CONFLICT BETWEEN THE USA AND CHINA AND AFTER THE COVID-19 PANDEMIC: WHO WILL BE THE WINNER AND WHO WILL BE THE LOSER?[1]

Introduction

The U.S. has been facing challenges to the economic superpower due to the rising power of China since 2010. After the economic reform in 1978 called the Open Policy, China's economic scale, foreign trade, and technological development have been growing rapidly. As a result, the Chinese economy became the second largest in the world in 2010, which was rather dramatic and happened very fast. As a result, China's role in the global economy has grown to be even more significant particularly since the global financial crisis (GFC) in 2008. It is widely recognized that the bilateral relationship between the U. S. and China will be a crucial determinant of the world's direction in the twenty-first century because China has tried to build a new form of cooperative platform in world politics and global economy by creating G2 in 2013 when President Xi, Jinping took the power (Hsieh, 2009; Kirton, 2013; Park, 2021; Xie, 2017).

In order to play its global roles properly in the global economy, China requested additional voting rights in the International Monetary Fund (IMF) in the G20 Summit of 2009, which would increase its political and decision-

---
[1] The research was financed from the project „Research on COVID-19" from the funds of the Adam Mickiewicz University, Poznan

making power within the IMF. In 2016, the Chinese currency, Yuan, officially joined the Special Drawing Rights (SDR) basket and became one of the foreign exchange reserve currencies of the IMF along with the U.S. Dollar, British Pound, Euro, and Japanese Yen. Although the Chinese voting rights in the IMF are still weaker than those of the U.S. and the EU, its economic power per se has already been the second-largest economy in the world since 2010. With the high economic growth of 6.1 percent in 2019, not only the U.S. but also the EU officially announced China to be an economic competitor in the pursuit of technological leadership and a systemic rival promoting the socialistic model of governance. The EU urged that China is no longer regarded as a developing country, but a key global actor and leading technological power. Therefore, China should take more responsibility for upholding the rules-based international order and greater reciprocity, non-discrimination, and openness of its system. In order to achieve it, Chinese publicly stated reform must be carried out into policies, and actions commensurate with its role and responsibility (Momani, 2016; IMF, 2015; European Commission, 2019).

With the rise of China as G2, it is significant to understand the bilateral trade relations between the U.S. and China and the impacts of the two nations' increasing interdependence on the global economy. Several negative perspectives on the trade conflicts between the U.S. and China had been already expressed in the mid of 2000s. The major reason for the proliferation of trade conflicts between the G2 was based on the U.S.'s large trade deficit with China that has led to a trade war between the two nations. As a result, it has weakened the bilateral trade relations between the G2 (Park, 2020).

Such a trend has continued through all of the U.S. presidencies and had led to protectionism since the Trump administration treated the trade conflicts as a trade war even though both parties are negotiating to solve the said trade conflicts. China has noticed fundamental changes in the U.S. government's stance regarding Chinese political and economic power. The U.S. considers China to be a serious threat to the U.S. global interests in all aspects. It also ruled out the possibility of China reforming gradually towards the Western system that resulted in a comprehensive review of past decades' U.S. policy towards China. Accordingly, the core reason for the trade conflicts between the two nations is not only the economy but also politics directed to gain global hegemony. This means that escalation of conflicts and confrontation is inevitable for the two nations (Chin et al., 2018; Zhang, 2019).

Since Jan. 2020, the world has been suffering from the COVID-19 pandemic, which has weakened the global economic growth and caused negative economic growth in most economies estimated by global economic institutions. Amid the pandemic, the trade war between the G2 has continued and most major economies have experienced economic and social lockdowns aimed to control the disease. Unfortunately, however, it is still an ongoing process and the global economy has a long way to overcome it although we expect a sharp economic rebound in 2021 (IMF, 2020; World Bank, 2020).

This paper argues when and why the trade conflict between the U.S. and China has started. It also analyzes what may be impacts of the trade conflict between the two economic superpowers as a whole and on the global economy in particular as well as how to solve the trade friction. Furthermore, it suggests possible measures how to prevent trade conflicts from U.S. protectionism in the future. Last, but not least, it also analyzes the economic impacts of the pandemic on G2. In order to find answers to these questions, critical analysis of literature, inference, and cross-sectional analysis based on statistical data are employed.

Theoretical debates

Most economists in the world would agree with recent rebuttals to skepticism about the liberal trading order because of widely and rapidly spreading protectionism around the world since the GFC in 2008. However, it is a fact that the intellectual and political support for free trade in the U.S. and elsewhere seems to have been weakened and protectionism has started ever since then even though G20 member nations agreed to prevent it at the G20 Summit in Washington D.C. Therefore, free trade based on multilateralism is regarded as wishful thinking for many countries particularly in the U.S. since the Trump administration.

The economic theory suggested comparative advantage and economies of scale would create economic gains through economic efficiency. Therefore, tariffs led to competitive tariff retaliation, which has resulted in a massive shrinkage in foreign trade and low global economic growth. Economic theory never claimed that free trade is good for all industries and all people. However, the winners from the free trade can afford to compensate the losers, and eventually, everyone could benefit because the aggregate gains are positive (O'Rourke and Williamson, 2001; Rosen, 2008).

Economic theory also states that resources will flow to more efficient uses. However, it does not apply when governments and markets do not work well. Therefore, Samuelson already urged in 1972 that the aggregate gains from trade are not necessarily positive for all nations. He expanded his idea further to claim that growth in the rest of the world can damage a country if it takes place in sectors that compete with its native exports that have a comparative disadvantage. As a result, a nation's relative and even absolute GDP per capita can fall in such a condition. Gomory and Baumol extended Samuelson's theory and stated that there is much possible equilibrium with vastly different outcomes for the countries involved in a modern free-trade world. They have further said that it is perfectly possible or rather common for a nation's equilibrium trade outcome to be less than the self-sufficiency outcome so that good equilibrium is often created rather than bestowed by nature. Accordingly, countries can do much to affect their trading outcomes. Therefore, they urge U.S. protectionism in trade (Samuelson, 2004; Gomory and Baumol, 2009).

However, Bhagwati criticizes Samuelson's explanation, saying that it cannot be used as a justification for U.S. protectionism. He also denies Gomory and Baumol's argument because the U.S. could not carry out effective industrial policies to remedy it although their argument is true. Krugman and Obsfeld support Bhagwati's critics that it is an empirical question rather than a fact whether the growth of emerging economies has indeed hurt advanced countries although theoretical possibility still exists (Bhagwati, 2009; Krugman and Obsfeld, 2009).

Economists have developed theoretical models for free trade and estimated welfare gains from reducing or eliminating trade barriers. In line with these models, Krugman, and Broda, and Weinstein suggested that trade benefits society through gains in overall quality and variety. However, this standard static growth from free trade has left trade promoters quite vulnerable because the static growth models consider only the short-run partial equilibrium efficiency gains. At the same time, the static models generate the gains from trade range very marginal (Krugman, 1997; Broda and Weinstein, 2006).

To deepen theoretical models finding long-term efficiency gains and contribution of free trade to economic growth, economists have developed dynamic models estimating impacts of trade liberalization used by cross-country regressions. By using these models, Bradford et al. urged that the U.S. economy in 2005 could generate higher economic growth than without post-war trade liberalization. However, Acemoglu left the issue of trade and growth undecided because there are models that highlight both positive and negative effects of trade on economic growth so that empirical work must be conducted. Accordingly, Lewer and Van den Berg pointed out that further development of dynamic models and additional empirical research is required. Additionally, linkages between trade and technology as well as trade and institutional quality must be further developed (Bradford, et al., 2006; Acemoglu, 2009; Lewer and Van den Berg, 2007; Feenstra et al., 2009).

In this paper, dynamic models rather than static models can be adopted because the former can explain the long-term benefits of free trade more precisely than the latter. Accordingly, the conservative dualism of trade theory explains why the U.S. protectionism has emerged since the GFC and it represents the trade policy of Trump and the U.K.'s conservative governments than any other theoretical background. However, it has limited to generate the global economic growth sustainability. Therefore, it is possible that the dynamic models based on long-term efficiency, in terms of gains and economic growth, can correct the direction of protectionism toward the free trade system based on multilateralism and the reciprocity principle.

Backgrounds and Reasons for Trade conflicts between the U.S. and China

The large size of the trade deficit between the U.S. and China has been a significant issue in bilateral trade relations since the mid of 2000s. The Trump administration regards the trade deficit with China as a significant sign of unfair Chinese economic policies. Therefore, it has reportedly requested China to develop a plan to reduce the bilateral trade deficit targeting by $ 100 billion. However, there is a large difference between the two nations' views on their official trade statistics. According to the U.S. trade statistics in 2017, the merchandise trade deficit with China accounted for $375.3 billion, while the Chinese trade surplus with the U.S. in the same year was $275.8 billion. Nearly $100 billion difference exists between the two nations that could cause a serious dispute between the two parties. Even though a statistical working group established by the U.S. – China Joint Commission on

Commerce and Trade (JCCT) in 2004 identified the causes of the statistical discrepancies, this does not mean any error in the official statistics of either country (Martin, 2018).

In fact, the U.S. has had the largest trade deficit in the world for over three decades since the 1970s. Exceptionally, the U.S. had briefly a trade surplus in the mid of 1970s but has experienced a continuous deficit since then. The U.S. deficit increased to over 5 percent of the national GDP in 2005 and fell to 2.9 percent of the national GDP in 2017, which started to decline slightly during the period of the Trump administration between 2017 and 2021. Owing to the rapid increase of the U.S.'s aggregate trade deficit, the Trump government criticized major U.S. trade partners in general and China in particular. The U.S. argues that China must correct its unfair trade policies, which generate huge trade surpluses and thus create trade imbalances between the two nations (Genereux, 2017; WTO, 2020; Park, 2020).

After over six decades-long free trade movements, the U.S. has shaken the foundations of the global trading system by imposing steep tariffs on imports from China and other major trading partners since President Trump took the power in 2017. The trade conflicts between the U.S. and other trading partners in general, and China in particular, started when the U.S. International Trade Commission (USITC) found that imports of solar panels and washing machines caused injury to the U.S. solar panel and washing machine industries in Oct. and Nov. 2017 respectively. Since then, G2 has imposed hostile tariffs on imports from both sides concerning manufacturing goods and even in technology and intellectual properties.

There are many reasons for trade conflicts whenever these take place regardless of nations and regions in which they occur. Among these, the trade conflict between the two major economies can be explained with the following four reasons that are claimed by the two parties commonly and observed by the outsiders. These are trade imbalance between the two nations, U.S. protectionism based on income inequality, China's unfair trade against intellectual property rights (IPRs), technology transfer and innovation for U.S. companies, and competition of hegemony power in the twenty-first century.

Firstly, the U.S. trade deficit with China accounted for $419 billion in 2018 that increased from $376 billion in 2017 although the Trump administration imposed high tariffs on imported goods from China. It declined to $ 346 billion and $284 billion in 2019 and 2020 respectively. The share of the U.S. trade deficit with China in 2018 accounted for nearly 42 percent of the total U.S. trade deficit although it declined from 49 percent in 2015. In fact, the share of the U.S. trade deficit with China has declined substantially since 2018. However, its share is still the highest (Amadeo, 2019; United States Census Bureau, 2020) (See fig. 1).

Secondly, the position of the U.S. as the largest economy in the world has led to protectionism since the GFC, in general, and the Trump administration, in particular, have impacted the global economies severely. U.S. protectionism hugely influences the global economy due to its economic size compared with other economies that result from the income inequality and distribution in the U.S. that has risen since the 2000s. Whatever the cause of the rise in inequality, the fact is that the average real wage of production per hour has been stagnant since the 1980s in the U.S. As a result, the wage increase in production has lagged behind the growth in real GDP per capita. Consequently, it has led the U.S. to be the second most unequal nation among OECD member nations based on the Gini index that increased up to 0.49 in 2018. (Krugman, 2009; ERP, 2009; Hillebrand et al., 2010; OECD, 2020; Alvaredo et al., 2017; www.statista.com, 2021).

Figure 1: The U.S. Trade Deficit with China from 2010 to 2020 (As of USD billion)

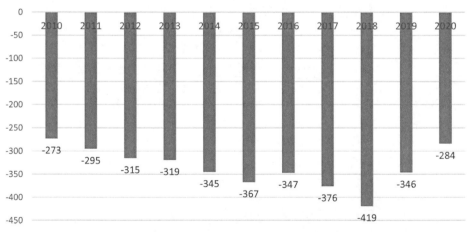

S o u r c e: United States Census Bureau, 2019 & 2020.

Thirdly, President Trump asked the U.S. Trade Representative (USTR) to investigate whether Chinese laws, policies, practices that may harm U.S. IPRs, innovation or technology development in Aug. 2017 or not, and the USTR initiated the investigation of China under Section 301 of the Trade Act of 1974. As explained earlier, it had found that China conducted unfair trade practices related to technology transfer, intellectual property, and innovation so that President Trump imposed 25 percent tariffs on 1,333 Chinese products in two phases starting July 2018. China also retaliated with an updated $50 billion list of 25 percent tariffs including agricultural and food products, crude oil, automobiles, airplanes, chemical products, medical equipment, and energy products, etc. (NG & Chung, 2018; USTR, 2018).

Last but not least, the U.S.-China trade conflict is based on the competition of a hegemony power in the twenty-first century. Therefore, several scholars expect that it would take a long term instead of a short term. In the national security strategy report in 2017, the U.S. called China its strategic rival. Additionally, the U.S. government specifically addressed a Chinese national development strategy, the Made in China 2025 program as a national threat in terms of high tech development that plays the core role in strengthening Chinese future competitiveness. In line with such a strategic point of view on the high tech area, President Trump signed the executive order to ban the Chinese high tech firms, Huawei in 2019, and TikTok as well as Weibo in 2020. Therefore, the key issue on the trade conflict between the U.S. and China is rather politics than economics that escalate confrontation between the two nations continuously in the future (The White House, 2017; Chin et al., 2018; Jiming, 2018; Doffman, 2019; BBC, 2020) (See table 1).

Table 1: Major Reasons for U.S. Protectionism

Reasons	Contents
Chronic U.S. trade deficit	The largest share of trade deficit to China up to 49 percent in total
High income inequality	Second highest Gini Index among OECD member nations Stagnant real wage since 1980
Chinese unfair trade practice	Violation of IPRs, technology transfer, etc.
Competition of global hegemony	Concerning the Made in China 2025 Program Technology ban to Chinese high tech firms: Huawei, TikTok, Weibo, etc.

S o u r c e: Author's adaptation

Who will be the Winner and the Loser from the Trade Conflicts and after the COVID-19 Pandemic?

The impacts of the trade conflict are not only bilateral but also multilateral and global. Particularly, the two largest economies in the world generate two-fifths of global GDP and about a quarter of global trade. Therefore, the bilateral trade conflict between G2 is highly worrisome for both the region and the world as the two nations are two of the three main hubs for global production chains (GPCs) and global value chains (GVCs) along with the European Union (EU) with tight trade links in key and various industrial sectors (Abiad et al., 2018; World Bank, 2020; WTO, 2020).

Most of the products affected in the bilateral tariffs imposed on imports of Chinese goods are mainly capital and intermediate goods that are targeted for the Made in China 2025 plan. In order to meet the target of the plan, China needs to import high-tech products for its end-products that are deeply connected with GVCs. On the contrary, China retaliated to impose tariffs mostly on imports of the U.S. agricultural products, chemicals, medical and energy equipment that are rather homogeneous goods available in the global markets. It means that China could face difficulties to import high-tech products from the U.S. or other advanced nations if the U.S. prohibits exporting these to China. In practice, the Trump administration has been banning high-quality semiconductor products using U.S. patents to be delivered to Chinese high-tech companies such as Huawei, SMIC, etc. since 2019 (Cerulus et al., 2020).

The second round of the trade conflict of $200 billion by the U.S. and $60 billion tariffs by China started in the mid of 2018 and had affected consumer goods as fewer supply chain lines were left to set the targets. The trade tension between the two nations has been continuously escalating and the U.S. threatened to impose tariffs of another $267 billion on Chinese imports, all of which all goods imported from China in 2018. China also threatened to retaliate with similar tariffs on all imports from the U.S. and considers other measures for retaliation to limit the U.S. FDIs and punish U.S. companies operating in China because the total import volume from the U.S. was much less than the total import from China. In the global trade tension, the U.S. government has considered setting the tariff of 25 percent on imports of automobiles and auto parts from all trading partners that would affect $350 billion worth of goods, which could impact the global economy severely and be the worst scenario imaginable. However, President Trump did not impose it and had been successively delaying it (Abiad et al., 2018; Park, 2018; Park, 2020).

The escalation of trade conflict and threats between the two economic superpowers caused a significant pressure of outlook for the global economic growth in general and the Chinese economy in particular. The Chinese export and sales started already weak in the third quarter of 2018 and continued to decline in 2019. Additionally, the threats influenced investors in the 'wait and see' mode and accelerated restrictions of foreign direct investment (FDI) for the high tech areas from China not only in the U.S. market but also in the EU market. As a result, Chinese economic growth declined from 6.9 percent in 2017 to 6.7 percent in 2018 and 6.1 percent in 2019 (Hanemann, 2018; State Administration of Foreign Exchange, 2019; World Bank, 2021).

In order to analyze the impacts of the trade conflict between the two nations on their economies, the implications of three scenarios are examined. The first scenario is a current scenario including all trade measures implemented as of Oct. 2018 with $200 billion of imports from China in 25 percent of tariffs. The second one is a bilateral escalation scenario intensifying to impose blanket tariffs of 25 percent on all merchandise imports from both countries. Finally, the last scenario is a worst-case scenario including measures under the bilateral escalation scenario and a global escalation of the trade conflict between the U.S. and other trading partners in automobiles and parts imposed by the U.S. on 25 percent tariffs of imports from other nations.

The immediate impact of these three scenarios will take time to be materialized fully. The current scenario was affected fully in 2019, while the direct impact of the worst scenario will be close to being in full effect in 2020 and completed in 2021. Moreover, the scenario modeling is used by the Asian Development Bank Multiregional Input-Output Table (ADB MRIOT) for the year 2017 to quantify the impact of changes in tariffs working through local and production chains that provides advantages in individual economies and sectors as well as understanding the structure and evolution of GVCs. The direct impact of the trade conflict is quantified at the product level gathered by published lists of tariff-affected commodities for all countries involved in the trade conflicts as of Sep. 2018. Additionally, these commodities are matched with detailed trade data from BACI and the United States Census Bureau in 2017 that uses a 6- to 10-digit Harmonized System Classification (Abiad et al., 2018; Wang et al., 2018).

Given the ADB analysis, the trade conflict between the two economies will be affected negatively in all scenarios. Under the current scenario, the Chinese economy would grow lower GDP by 0.48 percent, while the bilateral escalation scenario subtracts 0.55 percent GDP. In the worst-case scenario, the Chinese economic growth could be less by 1.05 percent. These impacts are based on direct, indirect, and trade redirection effects. On the contrary, the U.S. economy could be affected by the trade conflict less than the Chinese economy. It could subtract 0.12 percent, 0.08 percent, and 0.24 percent respectively. It indicates that the trade conflict can impact the two major economies rather marginal than expected in the midterm period although the Chinese economy could be affected more negatively than the U.S. economy. It may be the reason why the two nations carry trade conflicts without any hesitance continuously despite their agreement of trade deal in 2020 (See fig. 2).

Figure 2: Economic impact of the trade conflict on the U.S. and Chinese GDP by scenarios

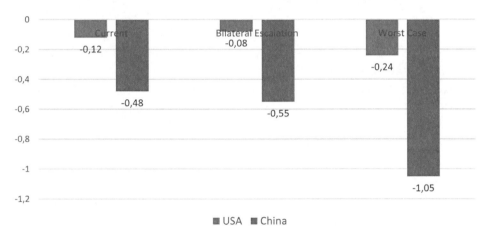

S o u r c e: Abiad et al., 2018.

Given the ADB analysis, the trade conflict between the two economies will be affected negatively in all scenarios even in the context world economy although it will affect the world economy less than the U.S. and Chinese economies as a whole. Under the current scenario, the global economy would grow lower GDP by 0.08 percent, while the bilateral escalation scenario subtracts 0.07 percent GDP. In the worst-case scenario, the global economic growth could be less by 0.25 percent. It shows that the trade conflict between the two major economies will impact the global economy nearly zero in the two scenarios, but affect very low in the worst-case scenario in the midterm period (Abiad et al., 2018).

However, some countries having a high trade dependence on China could be affected more severely than other countries. These countries are mostly

Asian countries such as Indonesia, Malaysia, South Korea, Singapore, Taiwan, Thailand, and Vietnam as well as Oceanian countries such as Australia and New Zealand. Particularly, Asian countries' exports of intermediate goods had been co-related closely with the global three economic blocs' industrial production index. These had more or less the same pattern between 2011 and 2019. It means that most Asian countries export their basic resources and intermediate goods to China and produce their final goods in China. Later, they export their final products to the EU and the U.S. markets (IMF, 2019).

Although the economic impact of the trade conflict on the global economy in the midterm could be marginal compared with those of the U.S. and China, it could threaten the collapse of the global production chains (GPCs) that have been built since the GATT in 1949. The GPCs are closely linked to the GVCs providing goods and services to the world market efficiently. The GPCs are composed of the three major production hubs such as China in Asia, Germany in the EU, and the USA in North America. If the GPCs in Asia are damaged, it would impact the other part of production hubs that could result in increasing production costs and creating unreliable global supply. As a result, it would damage the global supply chains (GSCs). It means that any damage to GPCs, GVCs, and GSCs could generate a further negative impact on global economic growth (Park, 2020; OECD, 2020).

In fact, the trade conflict will negatively impact the GPCs, GVCs, and GSCs in general and harm most of the Asian economies seriously, especially if it continues for longer and leads to the realization of the worst scenario. At the same time, some Asian countries such as Thailand and Vietnam could be benefited if multinational corporations (MNCs) move their production bases in China to these nations in order to overcome the U.S. high tariffs. However, the U.S. government has already noticed such a bi-effect and is ready to raise the tariffs on the products in these nations as well. As a result, the trade conflict could destroy the GPCs, the GVCs, and the GSCs in the long run if it is intensified (Abiad et al., 2018; Park, 2018; IMF, 2019).

This trend has been strengthened with the COVID-19 pandemic ever since Jan. 2020. The pandemic hit the Chinese economy first because the Chinese government started the lockdown process first in the world. As a result, most of the manufacturing activities stopped at the beginning of 2020. It caused the damage of the GPCs, GVCs, and GSCs severely so that many countries around the world were not able to produce their goods in time because parts and components produced in China could not be supplied as planned. Therefore, major economies such as the U.S. and the EU reconsidered to restore either their own GVCs and GSCs nearby or rebuild these new outside China. The U.S. in particular is keen to rebuild the new GVCs and GSCs with East Asian economic partners excluding China in the region to prepare the more resilient GVCs and GSCs in the post-COVID 19 era. Furthermore, the Japanese government has promoted to diversify GVCs by introducing a subsidy program either to relocate overseas production bases back to Japan or to construct strong supply chains involving ASEAN member countries to encourage transferring production bases from China (Lund et al., 2020; Urata, 2020).

As such some scholars and policymakers have suggested rethinking the GVCs by diversifying their supplier bases and reshoring activities because the subsequent lockdowns implemented all over the world could result in a GVC disruption, and the risks of that the re-nationalizing GVCs could to some extent insulate countries from the negative economic consequences of the Pandemic. However, some analytical work points out that the contraction of GDP would have been worse with re-nationalized GVCs because government lockdowns could also affect the supply of domestic inputs. Despite such various opinions on the GVCs with the pandemic, the common idea regarding COVID-19 and the GVCs is to strengthen the resilience of international production networks, to promote the security of supply, and mitigate disruptions in value chains (Baldwin, 2020; Bonadio et al., 2020; OECD, 2020).

The shift to more resilient and sustainable GVCs has been the core issue among government and business leaders in the time of COVID-19. The pandemic has catalyzed changes of GSCs that were already underway by promoting near-shoring and regionalizing of supply and production networks, extensive digitalization, and more sustainable production networks and practices. These efforts will bring more speed and flexibility to the GVCs and create closer GSCs than those existing before the COVID-19 pandemic on the global markets (De Nicola et al., 2020).

The global import intensity of production has reached its peak in 2008. Since the GFC in 2008, it showed a downturn trend despite a sharp rising from 2009 to 2011. Since then, the expansion of the GVCs has stopped and shown a declining pattern until 2019. It means that firms have reduced their use of foreign inputs and the GVCs have become shorter only in the international part. The reason for that is structural shifts such as the digitalization of economies, the servicification of manufacturing, and consumer preferences for more sustainable production processes. These are the main reasons why firms try to produce closer to consumers and rely less on offshoring while becoming more productive and providing better products and services. Additionally, there was also a concern about the consequence of trade tensions between G2 and rising protectionism worldwide that affected firms' higher trade costs and rising policy uncertainty (Miroudot & Nordström, 2019; OECD, 2020) (See fig. 3).

Figure 3: Global Import Intensity of Production (As of 1990 ~ 2019)

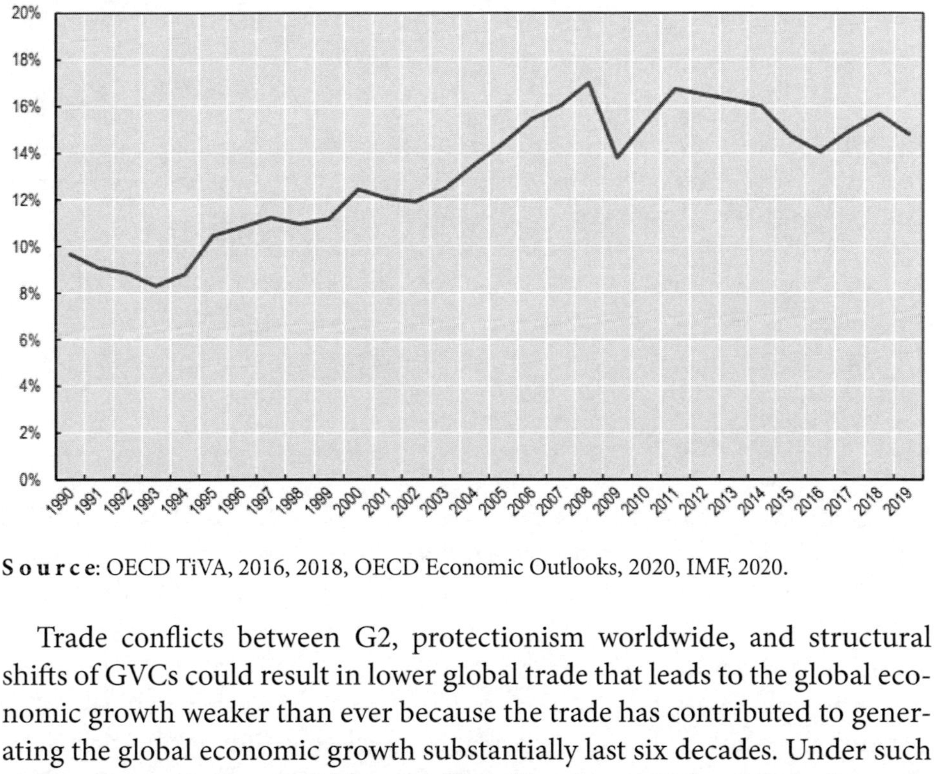

S o u r c e: OECD TiVA, 2016, 2018, OECD Economic Outlooks, 2020, IMF, 2020.

Trade conflicts between G2, protectionism worldwide, and structural shifts of GVCs could result in lower global trade that leads to the global economic growth weaker than ever because the trade has contributed to generating the global economic growth substantially last six decades. Under such circumstances, winners and losers affected by changing the global economic order will take place. Among the major and emerging economies, the winners are countries less dependent on trade for their GDP, while the losers are the countries with a higher dependency on trade because of their economic structures that are more vulnerable to the change of the global economic order. At the same time, the real losers are global consumers because they have to pay higher prices caused by higher tariffs and non-tariff barriers, which can decline the social welfare of the global consumers in general and technology development in particular (Park, 2018; Park, 2020) (See fig. 4).

Figure 4: Trade Dependency Ratio in GDP among Major and Emerging Countries (As of 2017, %)

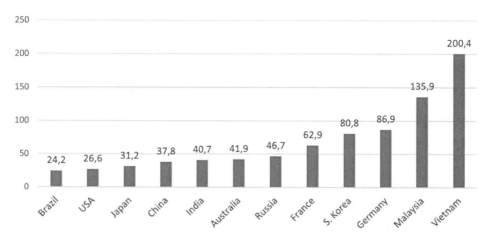

S o u r c e: https://en.wikipedia.org/wiki/List_of_countries_by_trade-to-GDP_ratio, 2021.

Conclusion

The trade conflict has always existed in the global economy that is rather common because some trading partners gain more benefit than others. In economic history, our lesson is that there are no winners from the trade conflict if it is not solved by dialogue, bilateral and multilateral trade agreements, but all economic actors become losers in the long run. We have already experienced the Great Depression in 1929/1930 that resulted in the Second World War that was the biggest tragedy of human being history in the twentieth century. Unfortunately, we are again experiencing severe trade conflicts between the two major economies in the twenty-first century, which may have a negative impact on the global economy if it continues without any proper solution put in place. Additionally, we are facing the COVID-19 pandemic causing the global economic downturn since 2020.

First of all, ironically, the trade conflict started from the U.S. pursuing trade protectionism particularly in the Trump administration having various internal problems such as trade imbalance with its trading partners, income inequality, etc. The U.S. government imposed high tariffs on imports of its trading partners. After revising KORUS FTA and NAFTA, the U.S. government focuses on the trade dispute with China and since 2017 it is still an ongoing process threatening to impose a 25 percent tariff on all import goods from China and vice versa. Furthermore, the U.S. government plans to impose a 25 percent tariff on the import of automobiles and parts from all countries although it has been delayed for six months in May 2019. Fortunately, it has not been imposed yet under the Trump administration, and the Biden administration starts in Jan. 2021. It is expected that the new U.S. government would take different approaches. At the same time, many specialists in global trade estimate that the Biden government will keep a hardline approach to China in terms of trade.

Since the severe trade conflict between the U.S. and China started in early 2018, several global and regional institutes such as IMF, ADB, European Central Bank (ECB) started to analyze the impacts of the trade conflict between the two major economies as well as the global economy. Additionally, individual nations' economic think tanks also joined this trend. For the impact of the trade conflict between the G2 on their national economies and the global economy in the midterm period, the analysis of most international economic institutions predicted a minor economic impact on the U.S. and China although the impact on China could be higher than that of the U.S. Additionally, the impact of the world economy could also be very low. It may be the reason why the two major economies are not afraid of continuing the trade conflict because the trade conflict could impact their economies marginal. Based on this reason, the trade conflict between the U.S. and China may continue at least in the midterm period if both parties are not satisfied with the outcome of their trade negotiation. Fortunately, the two nations agreed on the trade deal in Dec. 2019 and signed on it in Jan. 2020. However, many scholars suspect that the trade deal could not be implemented fully as planned. Since Jan. 2020, the global economy has struggled from the COVID-19 Pandemic and it is still passing the long channel in 2021.

Apart from the negative impact of the trade conflict on the G2 and the global economy, the most serious concern must be to damage the GPCs, the GVCs, and the GSCs due to the trade conflicts between the G2 and the COVID-19 pandemic, which will influence the global economy fundamentally in the longer term. These have been created since the GATT system and developed further through the WTO which is based on the free trade system. It has contributed to generating global economic growth last six decades. However, the global economic growth could be much lower than during the free trade era if these economic mechanisms for the GPCs, the GVCs, and the GSCs are damaged because of increasing production costs and insufficient flexibility, and uncertainty of trade policies. By changing the economic orders, many economies having high dependency rates in their GDP could be hit more negatively than other economies in the short term. Therefore, it is the only way to solve the trade conflict and the pandemic by reestablishing the free trade system based on multilateralism and the reciprocity principle for fair trade before all economic actors become the losers instead of becoming the winners in the long term.

References

Abiad A., Baris K., Bernabe J. A., Bertulfo D. J., Camingue-Romance S., Feliciano P. N., Mariasingham M. J., Mercer-Blackman V. (2018), *The Impact of Trade Conflict on Developing Asia*, "Asian Development Bank Economics Working Paper Series", No. 566, Dec., Manila: ADB.

Acemoglu D. (2009), *Modern Economic Growth, Princeton*, NJ: Princeton University Press.

Amadeo K. Y. (2019), *US trade Deficit with China and Why It's So High*, https://www.thebalance.com/u-s-china-trade-deficit-causes-effects-and-solutions-3306277, (accessed on 21 May 2019).

Baldwin R. (2020), *Supply Chain Contagion Waves: Thinking ahead on Manufacturing Contagion and Reinfection from the COVID concussion*, VoxEU.org, 1 April.

Bonadio B., Huo Z., Levchenko A., Pandalai-Nayar N. (2020), *Global Supply Chains in the Pandemic*, "NBER Working Paper", No. 27224.

BBC (2020), *US and China Sign Deal to Ease Trade War*, https://www.bbc.com/news/business-51114425, (accessed on 28 Dec. 2020).

Bhagwati J. (2009), *Does the U.S Need a New Trade Policy?* "Journal of Policy Modeling", Vol. 31, No.4.

Bradford S., Greico P., Hufbauer G. C. (2006), *The Payoff to America from Globalisation*, "The World Economy", Vol. 29, No. 7.

Broda C., Weinstein D. E. (2006), *Globalization and the Gains from Variety*, "The Quarterly Journal of Economics", Vol. 121, No. 2.

Cerulus L., Hendel J., Blatchford A. (2020), *How Biden Could Galvanize the World against Huawei?* "Politico", https://www.politico.eu/article/how-joe-biden-could-galvanize-the-world-against-huawei/, (accessed on 14 Jan. 2021).

De Nicola F., Timmis J., Akhlaque A. (2021), *How Is COVID-19 Transforming Global Value Chains? Lessons from Ethiopia and Vietnam*, https://blogs.worldbank.org/voices/how-covid-19-transforming-global-value-chains-lessons-ethiopia-and-vietnam, (accessed on 15 Jan. 2021).

Doffman Z. (2019), *Trump signs Executive Order That Will Lead to U.S. Ban on Huawei*, "Forbes", https://www.forbes.com/sites/zakdoffman/2019/05/15/trump-expected-to-sign-executive-order-leading-to-ban-on-huawei-this-week/#497d903168d9, (accessed on 23 May 2019).

European Commission (2019), *EU – China: A Strategic Outlook*, Strasbourg: EC.

Feenstra R. C., Mandel B. R., Reinsdorf M. B., Slaughter, M. (2009), *Effects of Terms of Trade Gains and Tariff Changes on the Measurement of U.S. Productivity Growth*, "NBER Working Paper", No. 15592.

Genereux F. (2017), *Protectionism: A Brake on Economic Growth*. "Economic Studies". https://www.desjardins.com/ressources/pdf/pv170217-e.pdf, (accessed on 20 Dec. 2020).

Gomory R., Baumol W. (2009), *Globalization: Country and Company Interests in Conflict*. "Journal of Policy Modeling", vol. 31, no 3.

Hsieh P. L. (2009) *China – United States Trade Negotiations and Disputes: The WTO and Beyond*, "Asian Journal of WTO and International Health Law and Policy", Vol. 4, No. 2.

International Monetary Fund (IMF) (2015), *IMF Executive Board Completes the 2015 Review of SDR Valuation*, Press Release No. 15/543, https://www.imf.org/en/news/articles/2015/09/14/01/49/pr15543, (accessed on 20 Dec. 2020).

International Monetary Fund (IMF) (2020), *World Economic Outlook: Growth Slow Down, Precarious Recovery*, 2020 April, (accessed on 09 Dec., 2020).

Jiming H. (2018), *China-US Trade Conflict: Causes and Impact*, "CF40-PIIE Joint Report", https://piie.com/system/files/documents/ha20180611ppt.pdf, (accessed on 23 May 2019).

Kirton J. (2013), *G20 Governance for a Globalized World*, Farnham: Ashgate.

Krugman P. R. (1997), *Increasing Returns, Monopolistic Competition, and International Trade*, "Journal of International Economics", Vol. 9, No. 4.

Krugman P. R., Obstfeld M. (2009), *International Economics*, Boston, MA: Pearson, Addison-Wesley.

Lewer J. J., Van den Berg H. (2007), *International Trade and Economic Growth*, Armonk, NY: M.E. Sharpe.

Lund S., Manyika J., Woetzel J., Barriball E., Krishnan M., Alicke K., Birshan M., George K., Smit S., Swan D., Hutzler K. (2020), *Risk, Resilience, and Rebalancing in Global Value Chains*, https://www.mckinsey.com/business-functions/operations/our-insights/risk-resilience-and-rebalancing-in-global-value-chains, (accessed on 15 Jan. 2021).

Martin M. F. (2018), *What's the Difference? – Comparing U.S. and Chinese Trade Data*, "CRS Report", RS 22640, Washington D. C.: CRS.

Miroudot S., Nordström H. (2019), *Made in the World Revisited*, "RSCAS Applied Network Science Working Paper" No. 2019/84, European University Institute.

Momani B. (2016), *China at the IMF*, in: Lombardi D., Wang H-Y, (eds.) Enter the Dragon: China in the International Financial System, Montreal & Kingston: McGill Queen's Press.

NG, T. and Chung, K. (2018), *Trade Conflict between China and the United States and Its Impact on Hong Kong's Economy*, Hong Kong: Research Office, Legislative Council Secretariat, https://www.legco.gov.hk/research-publications/english/1718in14-trade-conflict-between-china-and-the-united-states-and-its-impact-on-hong-kongs-economy-20180717-e.pdf, (accessed on 11. Dec. 2020).

Organization for Economic Cooperation and Development (OECD) (2014) *Fact Book 2014*, Paris: OECD.

Organization for Economic Cooperation and Development (OECD) (2020) *COVID-19 and Global Value Chains: Policy Options to Build More Resilient Production Networks*, http://www.oecd.org/coronavirus/policy-responses/covid-19-and-global-value-chains-policy-options-to-build-more-resilient-production-networks-04934ef4/, (accessed on 16 Jan. 2021).

O'Rourke K. H., Williamson J. G. (2001), *Globalization and History: The Evolution of Nineteenth Century Atlantic Economy*, Cambridge, MA: The MIT Press.

Park S–C (2018), *U.S. Protectionism and Trade Imbalance between the U.S. and Northeast Asian Countries*, "International Organizations Research Journal", Vol. 13, No. 2.

Park S-C (2020), *Trade Conflict Between the U.S. and China: What are the Impacts on the Chinese Economy?* "International Organizations Research Journal", Vol. 15, No. 2.

Park S-C (2021), *Asian Regional Cooperation: RCEP and CPTPP Strategy after Brexit*, in: Haba K. Holland M. (eds.) *Brexit and After: Perspectives on European Crises and Reconstruction from Asia and Europe*, Singapore: Springer.

Samuelson P. (2004), *Where Ricardo and Mill Rebut and Confirm Arguments of Mainstream Economists Supporting Globalization*, "Journal of Economic Perspectives", Vol. 18, No 3.

State Administration of Foreign Exchange (SAFE) (2019) *Annual Report of the State Administration of foreign Exchange 2019*, https://www.safe.gov.cn/en/file/file/20201221/6202b5b2b3834bafaa47fb7a5e81375b.pdf?n=Annual%20Report%20of%20the%20State%20Administration%20of%20Foreign%20Exchange%20(2019), (accessed on 14 Jan. 2021).

Strauss D. (2019), *Global Economy Counts Cost of Trade Dispute*, "Financial Times", 10 May.

The White House (2017) *National Security Strategy of the United States of America*, Washington D. C.: The White House, https://www.whitehouse.gov/wp-content/uploads/2017/12/NSS-Final-12–18–2017–0905.pdf, (accessed on 23 May 2019).

United States Census Bureau (2020), *Foreign Trade,* https://www.census.gov/foreign-trade/balance/c5700.html, (accessed on 21 Dec. 2020).

Urata S. (2020), *Reimagining Global Value Chains after COVID-19*, https://www.eria.org/news-and-views/reimagining-global-value-chains-after-covid-19/, (accessed on 15 Jan. 2021).

US Trade Representative (2018) *USTR Finalizes Tariffs on \$200 billion of Chinese Imports in Response to China's Unfair Trade Practices*, https://ustr.gov/about-us/policy-offices/press-office/press-releases/2018/september/ustr-finalizes-tariffs-200, (accessed on 23 Dec. 2020).

Wang Z., Wei S-J, Zhu K-F (2018), *Quantifying International Production Sharing at the Bilateral and Sector Levels,* "National Bureau of Economic Research Working Paper" No. 19677, https://www.nber.org/papers/w19677.pdf, (accessed on 25 Dec. 2020).

World Bank (2020), *World Bank Estimate*, https://data.worldbank.org/indicator/SI.POV.GINI?locations=US, (accessed on 22 Dec. 2020).

World Bank (2021), *World Bank Data*, https://data.worldbank.org/indicator/NY.GDP.MKTP.KD.ZG?locations=CN, (accessed on Jan. 14. 2021).

Xi J. P. (2017), *Secure a Decisive Victory in Building a Moderately Prosperous Society in all Respects and Strive for the Great Success of Socialism with Chinese Characteristics for a New Era*, Delivered at the 19th National Congress of the Communist Party of China, 18 October.

Zhang T. S. (2019), *China-US Strategic Competition: G1 or G2? China & US Focus*, April 30, https://www.chinausfocus.com/foreign-policy/china-us-strategic-competition-g1-or-g2, (accessed on Jan. 12. 2021).

Rafał Wiśniewski
Adam Mickiewicz University, Poznań
ORCID: 0000-0002-0155-246X

INTERNATIONAL LEADERSHIP, GREAT POWER COMPETITION, AND THE COVID-19 PANDEMIC – THE CASE OF SINO-AMERICAN RELATIONS[1]

The COVID-19 pandemic has proved to be a severe test of political institutions and governing mechanisms on all levels of human society. Authorities and leaders at all levels of government – local, national, regional, and global – have been faced with a crisis of scale, severity, and endurance rarely seen in recent memory. The successes and failures in managing this crisis will impact the legitimacy and, by extension, the future evolution of political institutions around the globe. The international order and its constituent institutions are not an exception. Due to its global scale and impact, the pandemic is a textbook example of a transnational threat, typical of the current era of deep and persistent globalization. It also provided a test of effectiveness for many institutions and arrangements meant to provide so-called global governance[2] within the existing international order. Moreover, this particular crisis has struck at a moment when this order was undergoing significant changes in the sphere of power distribution and international leadership. The competition between the two most powerful states – the U.S. and

---

[1] The research was financed from the project „Research on COVID-19" from the funds of the Adam Mickiewicz University, Poznan

[2] Global governance can be defined as "the totality of institutions, policies, norms, procedures and initiatives through which States and their citizens try to bring more predictability, stability and order to their responses to transnational challenges." (*Global governance and global rules for development in the post-2015 era*, 2014: vi)

the People's Republic of China – has intensified significantly becoming one of the crucial, if not the crucial issue on the global agenda, casting its shadow over all other international issues. This is mainly due to the fact, that the international position of the current order's leader – the U.S. – has weakened and PRC's claims to international leadership have strengthened. If such a transition of leadership would have taken place, it would mean a momentous shift in the shape and character of the international order. That is due to the fact that both states have quite different (often conflicting) visions concerning ordering international relations.

The pandemic may not be decisive for the changes mentioned above to take place. However, it has put both the U.S. and China at the center of the crisis and tested their merits as international leaders. Taking account of all these dynamics, this article aims to address the following research questions:
1. What are the effects of the pandemic on the international positions of both the U.S. and the PRC?
2. Did both powers' conduct in the course of the crisis strengthened or weakened their claims to the international leadership?
3. How the Pandemic can potentially influence the prospects of the U.S. and the PRC being the leader(s) of the future international order?

International order, international leadership, and great power competition.

Before we turn into a detailed analysis of the Sino-American competition for leadership in the international order and the way the pandemic impacts it, it is useful to shortly characterize the guiding concepts of this article – international order, international leadership, and great power competition.

We can start with the following characteristic of the international order: "(…) all political orders contain principles and norms that define how people and groups should behave towards each other, and all comprise arrangements for the exercise of power and the management of conflicts within, and between, particular collectives. Any political order rests on the distribution of power among its members: 'ordering' (that is, trying to govern) requires the capacity to influence the behavior of others, possibly even against resistance. Thus, any given order's specific characteristics reflect the ways in which the collective is governed. The international order spans all levels of governance, from the local to the global" (Maull, 2019: 9). Based on these assumptions we can think about the internal order as composed of three main elements: the actors (both state and non-state) and distribution of power among them; norms and rules guiding relations between them and institutions (including international organizations) which are meant to put these rules into practice and facilitate actors' cooperation. Actually, it can be argued that these constituent parts emerge in the exact sequence outlined above. The power dynamics taking place between actors of international relations lead to the emergence of particular rules and norms (the level of their specification and codification can vary greatly) which then serve as ideational foundations to build a functional institutional framework.

This is pretty much the way the current international order, which we can call the universalist liberal international order, came to being. After the Second World War, the United States emerged as the strongest power globally. This position gave it the means to realize ideas for political and economic order, guided by political values dominating its own political system, in the form of international legal and organizational structure (symbolized by, for example, United Nations, World Bank or General Agreement on Trade and Tariffs). Naturally, for four decades this order was far from global and universal. The Soviet Union had its own vision, which was in many respects a complete opposite of the U.S.-led order. Cold War can be understood as intense competition between these two visions for world order. After the collapse of the Soviet Union provided a definitive end to the Cold War, the American-led liberal order took hold globally, practically without serious competition.

Looking at the dynamic explained above, we can see that effective leadership is one of the crucial factors determining international order's survival and effectiveness. The author defines international leadership as one of the roles a state can play in the international community. Its effective exercise requires three elements: a strong position in the international hierarchy of power, a vision of international order and the will to realize it, and (last but not least) the acceptance of other actors. Power in international relations is a complex and often counterintuitive phenomenon (Baldwin, 2016). For the purpose of this article, it is enough to assume that an effective international leader needs to have a rich repertoire of power resources at its disposal. They include both material (GDP, financial reserves, technologies, military forces, etc.) as well as immaterial factors (the famous "soft power" or the proficiency and efficacy of its foreign policy machinery) which together give it the power, understood in relational terms ("an ability of A to make B do what A wants, even if it is against B's interests and/or will").

This is a good moment to pose the question of whether nation-states are the only actors of international relations capable of exercising international leadership? Although the influence and significance of numerous non-state actors have greatly increased in the last couple of decades, the power needed to lead the entire international order is still beyond their reach. Currently, nation-states are still institutions most capable to generate and mobilize power resources necessary for the said leadership and securing legitimacy for their use. The long-term research project organized by the German Institute for International and Security Affairs (SWP), which focused on the evolution of the international order since the end of the Cold War, concluded that state capacity is the most important factor influencing the effectiveness of the order. (Maull, 2019: 19) Based on that, we can safely assume that only the most powerful states in the system can effectively lead it. So international leadership is still pretty much the great-power game.

Power resources are a necessary condition for exercising international leadership, but, in itself, not a sufficient one. Playing the role of a leader in the international order entails having a vision of what values, norms and institutions should comprise it. Naturally, the level of detail can vary, and states rarely apply their stated values with absolute consistency. Nevertheless, the leader is supposed to influence the international agenda and offer solutions for the most pressing challenges facing the international community. Obviously, both the power resources and vision will not make an international leader out of a state whose leadership (and broader population) is not willing to play this role. American isolationism in the first half of the twentieth century is a case in point. The people's Republic of China has also long adhered to Deng Xiaoping's dictum of "keeping a low profile" (Yong Deng, 2008: 41), which led to assessments that it is unwilling to shoulder the responsibilities of leadership in the international community.

Finally, for a given state to exercise the leadership role, this needs to be accepted by others. To put it bluntly, a leader needs followers or at least supporters. Naturally, international leadership is rarely uncontested and it is difficult (if not impossible) to identify a threshold number of international actors, whose support guarantees the success of the leadership bid. We can assume that to count in this game, one needs to have a group of allies and/or partners. The size of this group is one of the factors determining whether we deal with a regional or global leader. For the purpose of this publication, we can simplify and claim that support of others for a given actor's international leadership can come from three main sources: coercion, calculation of benefits, and attractiveness. All of the three have some role to play and in various circumstances, different motivations can prove decisive. However, it can be argued that successful international leadership rests on a mix of all three factors. Different forms of coercion (military or economic) are sometimes required to enforce norms and otherwise police (safeguard) the order. Naturally, it is almost impossible to base leadership of the international order entirely on coercion. Other actors need to see some benefits for themselves. Here the other two factors come into being. International order and its leader(s) can be considered legitimate when it delivers what we can call "international public goods". It is a broad category that includes such things as security guarantees, profits from international economic interactions, stability, predictability, practical cooperation, access to resources, international infrastructure, etc. One of the international leader's responsibilities is to provide such goods to other members of the international community. Finally, the sheer attractiveness of the leader's vision and other aspects of broadly understood "soft power" can help to legitimize the leadership position.

To understand the leadership dynamics in the current international order it is important to look at its post-Cold War evolution. After the Soviet Union's collapse, the U.S.'s position as the only superpower has enabled the near-universal (if sometimes grudging) acceptance of the universalist liberal international order and Washington's leadership within it. Other great powers either shared the American vision of international order and supported the U.S. leadership (like the UK, France, or Japan) or held their reservations but stopped short of full-blown contestation and pushback (like the PRC and Russian Federation). Enormous American power advantage made a successful counter-bid for global leadership very difficult. However, at the turn of the twenty-first century's first and second decade, the character and substance of great power relations have undergone a significant shift. The financial crisis and costly military interventions in the Greater Middle East have degraded both the power position and international prestige of the United States. At the same time, PRC's power has been consistently growing, making this state a viable contender for the position of the second superpower. At the same time, both Russia and China (independently and sometimes in coordination) increased their contestation of the liberal international order and challenged American leadership in connection to a series of crises (Ukraine, Syria, South China Sea). It can be argued that during the last decade the nature of Sino-American relations changed from both actors being simply competitors in the global game for position and influence into full-blown rivals, perceiving each other as threats to their most vital national interests. (Poast, 2020)

The importance of this change for the topic of this article is hard to understate. In the first two decades following the end of the Cold War, relations between great powers experienced a radical shift in favor of cooperation. Sources of tension or outright conflicts didn't disappear completely. However, practically all great powers of the time accepted (sometimes only partially) the broad outline of the liberal international order and shared similar development strategies (based on growing integration with the global economy). Erik Gratzke described this trend as a "capitalist peace." According to him three elements made developed capitalist economies unlikely to engage in war against one another: 1) rising importance of financial and intellectual capital making territorial expansion less profitable 2) overlap of foreign policy goals of developed nations 3) rise of capital markets creating new mechanisms of competition and communication (Gartzke, 2007). This economic interdependence was accompanied by a political reality of most great powers being affected by a shared set of transnational (or global) problems, including environmental degradation, financial crisis, infectious diseases, terrorism, etc. which can realistically be tackled (or rather managed) only by cooperation (Shunji Cui and Buzan, 2016).

A global pandemic of a highly infectious disease is just the type of threat that great powers of the post-Cold War period would be expected to cooperate in tackling. However, the growing animosity, (or even hostility) between the current international order's greatest powers (the U.S. and the PRC) has slowly but visibly shredded the fabric of post-Cold War consensus and cooperation (however imperfect it had been). During Donald Trump's term in office, this growing tension very publicly burst into the open. Starting with the 2017 National Security Strategy the U.S. government has openly named China as a "strategic competitor. (*National Security Strategy of United States of America*, 2017: 2–3) The United States Strategic Approach to The People's Republic of China, published by the White House in May 2020, clearly states that: "Given the strategic choices China's leadership is making, the United States now acknowledges and accepts the relationship with the PRC as the CCP has always framed it internally: one of great power competition." (United States Strategic Approach to The People's Republic of China, 2020: 8)

To summarize, the current global crisis provoked by the pandemic has struck at a potentially critical juncture in the evolution of the international order. Exactly at the moment when effective international leadership has been needed and expected, the two greatest powers have been engaged in escalating competition for power and prestige. This definitely complicated the international response and arguably (partially) paralyzed the institutional framework of international cooperation. (Patrick, 2020)

The Pandemic as a test of international leadership credentials.

After establishing what international leadership entails and painting the picture of current Sino-American rivalry in that regard, we can now discuss whether any of the contestants have actually displayed the required abilities during the global crisis caused by COVID-19. Looking at the definition of international leadership outlined in the previous section, we can assume that the international community expected the state playing that role to show three attributes (sub-roles):

a) **Role-model** – to lead the world in such a challenging time, a state would be expected to demonstrate that it is able to deal with the threat effectively within its borders and thus provide examples of good practices to other members of the international community.

b) **Convener/coalition builder** – as the chief architect and enforcer of the international order, the leading power would be expected to organize and coordinate the international response to the crisis. In the case of a pandemic, this would entail empowering existing institutions (primarily the World Health Organization – WHO) and/or building ad hoc coalitions and initiatives to deal with emerging problems (like joint development of vaccines, economic aid, distribution of medication, etc.).

c) **Provider of public goods** – the leading power would also be expected to provide meaningful aid to other states (primarily allies) which would include financial support, medicine and medical equipment, medical personnel, etc.

Did the U.S. and/or China successfully played any of these roles in the Pandemic thus far? Let's start with the incumbent international leader – United States. In all three respects listed above, America proved to disappoint expectations. With regards to the effectiveness of its response to the crisis, the overwhelming public image around the world was rather of the U.S. federal government as being an anti-role model of successful pandemic response. Chaotic policy decisions, soaring numbers of infections and fatalities, visible disregard of large segments of the public for preventive measures, all accompanied and topped by presidential rhetoric belittling the scale of the crisis, all contributed to an image of a slow-motion catastrophe rather than a competently planned and efficiently executed response. (Johnson, 2020) All this was very visible to the international audience due to the media and political environment permissive of rolling and critical media coverage. When it comes to leading the international response to the pandemic, the policy of Donald Trump's administration had also underachieved. It is true that border closures and sometimes aggressive acquisition of medical supplies for one's own needs proved to be rather widespread practices across the international community. However, the very public indifference or even hostility of the incumbent superpower's government towards the primary international institutions tasked with confronting the crisis (primarily the WHO, but also the COVAX vaccine alliance) seemed to be a direct opposite of what the leader of the international order would be supposed to do (Patrick, 2020). The U.S. government proved to be quite uninterested in organizing and coordinating a coherent international response to the Pandemic. This is also related to the third aspect of international leadership under discussion – the provision of public goods. According to official data, by August 2020 different agencies of the U.S. federal government committed approximately 1.6 $bn to aid other countries in dealing with COVID-19 (Moss, Oum and Kates, 2020). However, numerous voices in the public debate questioned the real scale and efficiency of American international aid in this area (Anna, 2020; Igoe, 2020).

It is difficult to directly compare the actual financial and material contributions of both powers to countering pandemic beyond their borders (in no small part due to limited official Chinese data on the matter (Kurtzer, 2020). Two things however stand out. First, considering America's position as the current international leader and its past record of assistance and public goods' provision the scale and tempo of its response may seem underwhelming (Runde, Savoy and McKeown, 2020). Second, China has publicized its assistance relentlessly, painting a convincing image of an engaged and (arguably) generous donor (Kao and Li, 2020; Schrader, 2020). To summarize, the U.S. was not very successful in fulfilling expectations concerning its leadership in fighting the pandemic.

Did the international leader's mantel fit China better? When thinking about international perceptions of Beijing's handling of the pandemic it is important to distinguish two phases. After the outbreak of the new virus in Wuhan became public knowledge, Chinese authorities have been heavily criticized for a slow response and lack of transparency concerning the origins and scale of the disease. This created a very serious threat to China's positive image around the world. It is admittedly hard to claim the role of an international leader when a strong narrative in the global public debate assigns responsibility (or even culpability) for the pandemic to your state. Significant doubts about the adequacy and sincerity of the initial response in the PRC persisted consistently (Page and Khan, 2020; *China delayed releasing coronavirus info, frustrating WHO*, 2020). However, this situation quickly changed. As the local epidemic turned into a pandemic, other states (including the U.S.) turned out to be even less prepared for the crisis. Relatively quickly the narrative concerning the crisis response turned in China's favor. Later stages of Chinese mitigation measures proved to be very effective (even if draconian from the perspective of citizen rights). At the same time, the majority of states around the world (including advanced Western democracies leading the current international order) proved incapable of taming the crisis accordingly. Detailed comparative analysis of various national strategies to counter the pandemic goes beyond the scope of this article. What is important at this point, is the fact that the overwhelming public perception was one of the highly effective Chinese measures comparing very favorably with Western power's sometimes chaotic and ineffective approach. In consequence, it can be claimed that PRC has been relatively successful in demonstrating leadership by being a model of effective pandemic response. However, this success is not without caveats, which concern persistent doubts about the PRC authorities' responsibility for early missteps and suppressing information about the outbreak when the rest of the world needed it most.

When it comes to China's role in coordinating global response and providing public goods the preliminary record is also mixed. PRC has not actively launched new international initiatives aimed at tackling the pandemic. However, it deftly capitalized on public U.S. indifference (or outright hostility) towards international institutions. When the Trump administration withdrew from WHO, president Xi Jinping very publicly pledged additional donations to the organization. China also joined the COVAX initiative, which has been shunned by America. Looking at the implication for the leadership dynamic within the international order, such moves can be viewed as scoring easy diplomatic points through exploiting competitors' weaknesses. However, it is difficult to argue that China has fully adopted the role of coordinator of the global response to COVID-19.

Chinese international activity proved to be the biggest and most visible in the area of medical aid. It is difficult to find precise data about the scale of financial contributions made by Beijing towards combating the pandemic (Kurtzer, 2020). However, it is beyond doubt, that PRC offered significant assistance in terms of medical personnel and equipment to many states around the world (as of May 31, 2020, China had sent 29 medical expert teams to 27 countries, and offered assistance to 150 countries and 4 international organizations (*Fighting COVID-19: China in Action*, 2020). This assistance was understandably welcomed and needed. It was also intensely publicized by Chinese state media and diplomacy to impress on audiences (both domestic and foreign) the image of the PRC as a responsible power, extending assistance to those who need it most. However, the entire effort didn't prove to be uncontroversial. Some countries registered serious complaints about the quality and reliability of equipment manufactured in China (it is important to note, however, that the most publicized cases this related to commercially purchased items, not those provided as part of official Chinese state aid (Dudik and Tomek, 2020; *Coronavirus: Countries reject Chinese-made equipment*, 2020). In other cases, the conduct of Chinese diplomats proved to generate controversies. The actions which generated concerns included pressure on public expressions of gratitude and crushing public rebuke to any criticism of China's actions. It can be argued that this combative style in Chinese diplomacy (often called "Wolf Warrior diplomacy") neutralized a sizable part of goodwill generated by Beijing's aid efforts (Kang, 2020).

It is a paradoxical situation when a huge chance for improving China's public image around the world has been partially wasted by diplomatic assertiveness. In this context, it is also important to note the case of further deterioration in PRC's relations with Australia. When Australian prime minister Scott Morrison supported the notion of an independent international inquiry into the virus's origins, Beijing responded by cutting a significant portion of Australian exports to China, with not really veiled intent of punishing this perceived insult. This lead to the strengthening of the "sinoskeptic" sentiment in Australia (Karp and Davidson, 2020; *The Economist*, 2020). What can explain this paradoxical messaging to the world by China's leaders? This author believes that an important part of the explanation concerns the prime audience of the Chinese propaganda efforts. Although its authors clearly intended to impress the foreign audience, the main target was the domestic population. The core aim of state policy in PRC is to maintain the power of the Communist Party. In this context, the propaganda push accompanying medical aid to other countries was primarily meant to convince the Chinese public, that the Party is admired around the world for its effective handling of the crisis and the aid it extended to foreigners. In this context, harsh diplomatic language can be perceived as defending the good name of the country.

To summarize, looking at the record from 2020 alone, it can be argued that China was rather more successful than the U.S. in fulfilling expectations of international leadership during the pandemic. However, Beijing's success in this regard is far from complete. It is more relative (contrasted with the failure of the U.S. leadership) than absolute. The PRC has not taken a very active role in coordinating the international response to COVID-19. Additionally, huge potential gains in prestige and goodwill, made possible by medical aid, have been partially contradicted by the assertive defense of national interests (good name among them).

Future leadership prospects

In this section, we will look at the pandemic's consequences for the ability of both the U.S. and the PRC to fulfill an international leadership role in the short- and medium-term future. To that end, three factors necessary to fulfill this role (mentioned earlier in the article) will be analyzed – power position, the vision of international order, and allies.

Pandemic's effects on both states' power position are mostly a product of its economic effects. How their economies will weather disruption caused by COVID-19 will determine the scale of material resources available for their bilateral competition in many spheres. Preliminary assessments of postpandemic economic prospects are far from positive. According to the calculations made by *The Economist* (based partially on World Bank data), the output lost due to the pandemic in 2020 amounts to $1.7trn and $680bn in China (*The Economist*, 2021). What is clear, is that all economies will come out of the crisis weakened. However, it seems that the U.S. economy has suffered bigger losses in output, jobs, and investment than the Chinese. China is practically the only big economy that returned to GDP growth in 2020. Its short to medium-term growth prospects seem to be better than America's. Several prognoses now assume that China's GDP will overcome America's in this decade (earlier than originally envisioned) (Elliot, 2020; Uehara and Tanaka, 2020). Naturally further the wellbeing of the Chinese economy is not guaranteed, there are also risk factors concerning foreign and domestic demand or indebtedness.

Potential economic consequences of the pandemic have implications for other dimensions of state power as well. Already before COVID-19 struck, there were serious doubts about America's ability to keep pace in power competition with China. Blankenship and Denison argue that the U.S. was able to sustain Cold War rivalry with the Soviet Union in no small part due to mobilization of fiscal resources for military and R&D spending. Currently, although the American economy is significantly bigger than it was during the Cold War years, changes in the political economy resulted in the state being able to command a smaller share of it (Blankenship and Denison, 2019). The post-pandemic economy and state will probably be even more challenged to provide resources for such a competition. Some observers already foresee stagnation or even cuts in defense expenditure (Barno and Bensahel, 2020). It is also important to note that economists predict that post-pandemic economic hardship will hit the socio-economic pressure points of Western economies even further, probably increasing social and political pressures challenging the political establishment and increasing political instability (Reinhart and Reinhart, 2020).

Now we can turn to the second factor of successful international leadership – the vision of international order. Leaders of both the U.S. and the PRC have clear ideas on what rules should guide international politics and they considerably diverge from one another. They can be summed up as universalist liberal order (promoted and led by the U.S.) and multipolar order of national particularities (promoted by China). The main points of both visions can be summarized in the following way. The universalist liberal order is meant to be based on the strong leadership of the dominant superpower (the U.S.). As the name implies, it is based on norms, values, and ideas derived from liberal political and economic thought. It is meant to promote and defend these ideals. These include both transforming domestic political and economic institutions of its members and effective enforcement of norms through a formalized institutional structure. The universalism of this vision manifests itself in both openness to all willing actors and the universal character of norms, values, and ideas underpinning it. The vision of a multipolar order of national particularities, by contrast, stresses the existence of multiple independent power centers, without the necessary hegemony of one particular leader. It is meant to protect the diversity of political and economic models. Its central values are sovereignty and non-interference in members' domestic affairs. For that reason, its institutional framework is less formalized and there is less emphasis on rules' enforcement. Finally, in contrast to liberal vision's universalist ambitions, it postulates a particular character of cooperation.[3]

Has the experience of the pandemic influenced the attractiveness of these visions for the global public? It is important to note, at this point, that the actually realized universalist liberal order has been undergoing a serious crisis for some time before the pandemic struck. This can be traced at least to the global financial crisis (2007–2009). Two main factors undermined the operation and support for this order: the rise of illiberal states and the crisis of liberalism in Western countries. In this sense, the order has been contested both from the outside (by authoritarian powers contesting its rules and offering some alternatives) and from within (by the rise of anti-establishment sentiments and political parties leading to erosion of liberal norms and adoption of illiberal policies) (Cooley and Nexon, 2020; Boyle, 2020). Naturally, the same factors have strengthened the appeal of the Chinese vision of the multipolar order of national particularities. The discourse surrounding responses to the pandemic strengthened the case of viewing nation-states as the institution of security provision and reinforced the notions of safeguarding sovereignty and autonomy. All of this, coupled with the perceived ineptitude of Western liberal democracies in handling the pandemic, might further undermine the legitimacy of the universalist liberal order. However, it should also be noted that increased (and very public) oppressiveness of the Chinese state towards its citizens (visible in the repression of Uighurs or limitation of Hong Kong's autonomy) has created very negative publicity and genuine opposition from many audiences around the world (Silver, Devlin and Huang, 2020). Naturally, this was most visible in democracies, but this may point out towards longevity of liberal ideas.

Finally, we will consider the effects of the current crisis on the alliance relationships of both contestants for international leadership. It might be argued that the pandemic didn't really alter the trajectories visible before

---

[3] The competing visions of international order are explained and analyzed in detail in author's previous publications - (Wisniewski, 2019) (Wisniewski, 2020: 90–109).

its onset. The U.S. enjoys a big advantage over the PRC thanks to its long-standing and rich pool of allies and partners. Although China has enjoyed good relations with many states, it is difficult to identify genuine allies, fully supporting its foreign policy. Potentially the most valuable development of the last decade is the strengthened cooperation with Russia, following Moscow's fallout with the West over the war in Ukraine. However, it is important to remember that the assertive and sometimes chaotic policy of the Trump administration has led to a sense of crisis in the U.S. alliance system. That is visible both in Europe and Asia. The new administration of Joe Biden declares repairing this damage to be its foreign policy priority. Its success is highly dependent (among other factors) on whether allied capitols see Trump's term as an anomaly, or whether assessments of America's reliability as an ally changed more profoundly. In the case of the PRC, it is difficult to identify states which tilted towards China on a strategic level during the pandemic. China's assertive style (described earlier) was one of the contributing factors.

To summarize, it seems that the pandemic has mainly strengthened the trends already visible in the leadership dynamic of the international order. America's material power and ideo-political appeal weakened visibly. Beijing seems to be well-positioned to capitalize on this, but the sufficient power (and crucially) international support still seems not fully adequate for an effective leadership bid.

Conclusions

Throughout this article, the author has presented his analysis of the ways in which the COVID-19 pandemic has tested the U.S. and Chinese international leadership credentials and their future prospects. The global health crisis struck at the moment when American leadership of the international order had been weakening. All its pillars – material power, ideological vision, and international relationships - although still very strong, had been very perceptively on a mildly declining (or stagnating) trajectory. China meanwhile, was in a relatively good position to translate its rapidly growing power into a successful leadership bid. At the same time, Beijing faced important domestic and international constraints on fully realizing this potential. The pandemic crisis seems to have strengthened these trends. It further sapped trust in American leadership and contributed to the erosion of U.S. material capabilities. At the same time, Beijing's seeming success in coping with the pandemic seemed to increase its power and appeal. However, so far, Beijing didn't prove decisively successful in widely convincing the international community to share and support its vision of global leadership.

In terms of prognosis, the author would like to propose four scenarios, withholding judgment on relative probabilities of their realization.

1. **China as the new leader** – it is possible that the trends outlined in this text will continue to strengthen the PRC's power position and the attractiveness of its vision for the international order. In this scenario, the erosion of the U.S. power and prestige would continue, probably accompanied and strengthened by the growing dysfunction of the U.S. political system. If simultaneously, China would be able to maintain its political stability and sustain economic growth, it could end up in a position of being the role-model and provider of public goods. Naturally, that would require the sustained determination of the party-state leadership to push for active engagement and assuming leadership position within the international order. In this case, the Pandemic could act as another catalyst of the relative U.S. decline and Chinese ascendancy.

2. **America resurgent** – In this scenario, the U.S. would be able to renew the sources of its leadership and maintain its dominant position in world affairs. Such a scenario would require overcoming significant challenges in terms of reinvigorating the economy, overcoming the dysfunctional tendencies within the domestic political system, and reassuring allies around the world that America is both able and worthy to continue its leadership. Such an outcome would have been added by Beijing's ineptness in convincing global audiences to support its political vision and in building lasting partnerships/alliances.

3. **A world divided (new Cold War)** – It is also conceivable that both powers will maintain strong material, the ideational and political basis for international leadership, but insufficient to assume the position of truly global dominance. This scenario also assumes that the Sino-American relationship will continue to be very antagonistic. That could lead to the emergence of two blocks within the international community – one "liberal" under the U.S. leadership and the second "sovereignist/authoritarian" under the PRC's leadership. Such a situation might be plausible, considering the fact that backlash against Chinese assertiveness and repressive politics (outlined earlier in the article) is highly concentrated in

democratic (largely Western) states. It can be argued that many developing countries might be more open to the Chinese leadership. In this context, it is interesting to note the opinion of John Prideaux (the U.S. editor for The Economist) that the Chinese challenge may reinvigorate the idea of the West as a cohesive political block. (Prideaux, 2020) The gradual build-up of two alternative techno-spheres is another indicator pointing in that direction.

4. **Zero-polar world**. This scenario assumes that domestic social, economic, and political challenges, catalyzed by the pandemic, could lead both the U.S. and the PRC to turn inwards and ease their push towards international leadership. In such a case we might see the realization of a "zero-polar world" scenario. It essentially means that no actor has the power and (crucially) the will to take active leadership (and responsibility) for maintaining the global order (Manning, 2013: 120–122). Already we can see the trends which make such a scenario imaginable. The new Biden administration is clearly focusing on domestic priorities concerning the pandemic response, economic recovery, and dealing with internal division in the American society. For Beijing, managing the short- and medium-term economic and social effects of the pandemic will also most certainly prove quite absorbing. This scenario does not envision the U.S. and China withdrawing from their competition in some form of isolationism. Rather it assumes that ambitious foreign policy goals (including international leadership) will take second place to domestic priorities. If that would come true, it would mean that a leadership vacuum would appear in the international system. One possible variant of this scenario can include other great powers (i.e. European powers/EU, India, Japan, etc.) stepping in and trying to fill at least a part of this vacuum. However, considering that these actors face similar challenges and face considerable power constraints, the prospect of a new leadership configuration seems moderate at best.

References

Anna C. (2020), *Aid groups 'alarmed' by little US coronavirus assistance*, Associated Press. Available at: https://apnews.com/article/e8502c6c8556ed5ff-3ca84e48b198753 (Accessed: 9 February 2021).

Baldwin D. A. (2016), *Power and International Relations. A Conceptual Approach.* Princeton: Princeton University Press.

Barno D., Bensahel N. (2020), *Five Ways the U.S. Military Will Change After the Pandemic, War On The Rocks.* Available at: https://warontherocks.com/2020/04/five-ways-the-u-s-military-will-change-after-the-pandemic/ (Accessed: 9 February 2021).

Blankenship B. D., Denison B. (2019), *Is America Prepared for Greatpower Competition?*, "Survival", 61(5).

Boyle M. J. (2020), *America and the Illiberal Order After Trump,* "Survival", 62(6).

China delayed releasing coronavirus info, frustrating WHO (2020) *Associated Press.* Available at: https://apnews.com/article/3c061794970661042b18d5aeaaed9fae (Accessed: 9 February 2021).

Cooley A., Nexon D. H. (2020), *How Hegemony Ends,* "Foreign Affairs", 99(4).

Coronavirus: Countries reject Chinese-made equipment (2020) "BBC News". Available at: https://www.bbc.com/news/world-europe-52092395 (Accessed: 9 February 2021).

Cui S., Buzan B. (2016), *Great power management in international society,* "Chinese Journal of International Politics", 9(2), pp. 181–210. doi: 10.1093/cjip/pow005.

Deng Y. (2008), *China's Struggle for Status The Realignment of International Relations.* Cambridge: Cambridge University Press.

Dudik A., Tomek R. (2020), *Faulty Virus Tests Cloud China's European Outreach Over Covid-19, Bloomberg.* Available at: https://www.bloomberg.com/news/articles/2020–04–01/faulty-virus-tests-cloud-china-s-european-outreach-over-covid-19 (Accessed: 9 February 2021).

Elliot L. (2020), *China to overtake US as world's biggest economy by 2028, report predicts,* "The Guardian", 26 December. Available at: https://www.theguardian.com/world/2020/dec/26/china-to-overtake-us-as-worlds-biggest-economy-by-2028-report-predicts.

Fighting COVID-19: China in Action (2020). Available at: http://english.scio.gov.cn/whitepapers/2020–06/07/content_76135269.htm.

Gartzke E. (2007), *Capitalist Peace,* "American Journal of Political Science", 51(1).

Global governance and global rules for development in the post-2015 era (2014). Available at: https://www.un.org/en/development/desa/policy/cdp/cdp_publications/2014cdppolicynote.pdf.

Igoe M. (2020), *What's behind the backlash against a White House pandemic proposal?, Devex.* Available at: https://www.devex.com/news/what-s-behind-the-backlash-against-a-white-house-pandemic-proposal-97996 (Accessed: 9 February 2021).

Johnson M. (2020), *The U.S. was the world's best prepared nation to confront a pandemic. How did it spiral to "almost inconceivable" failure?,* "Milwaukee Journal Sentinel", 14 October. Available at: https://eu.jsonline.com/in-depth/

news/2020/10/14/america-had-worlds-best-pandemic-response-plan-play-book-why-did-fail-coronavirus-covid-19-timeline/3587922001/.

Kang D. (2020), *China's Diplomats Show Teeth in Defending Virus Response*, *The Diplomat*. Available at: https://thediplomat.com/2020/04/chinas-diplomats-show-teeth-in-defending-virus-response/ (Accessed: 9 February 2021).

Kao J., Li M. S. (2020), *How China Built a Twitter Propaganda Machine Then Let It Loose on Coronavirus*, *ProPublica*. Available at: https://www.propublica.org/article/how-china-built-a-twitter-propaganda-machine-then-let-it-loose-on-coronavirus (Accessed: 9 February 2021).

Karp P., Davidson H. (2020), *China bristles at Australia's call for investigation into coronavirus origin*, "The Guardian", 29 April. Available at: https://www.theguardian.com/world/2020/apr/29/australia-defends-plan-to-investigate-china-over-covid-19-outbreak-as-row-deepens.

Kurtzer J. (2020), *China's Humanitarian Aid: Cooperation amidst Competition*, *Center for Strategic and International Studies*. Available at: https://www.csis.org/analysis/chinas-humanitarian-aid-cooperation-amidst-competition (Accessed: 9 February 2021).

Manning R. A. (2013), *US Strategy in a Post-Western World*, "Survival", 55(5).

Maull H. W. (2019), *The Once and Future Liberal Order*, "Survival", 61(2).

Moss K., Oum S., Kates J. (2020), *U.S. Global Funding for COVID-19 by Country and Region*, *Kaiser Family Foundation*. Available at: https://www.kff.org/global-health-policy/issue-brief/u-s-global-funding-for-covid-19-by-country-and-region/ (Accessed: 9 February 2021).

National Security Strategy of United States of America (2017). Available at: https://www.whitehouse.gov/articles/new-national-security-strategy-new-era/.

Page J., Khan N. (2020), *On the Ground in Wuhan, Signs of China Stalling Probe of Coronavirus Origins*, "The Wall Street Journal", 12 May. Available at: https://www.wsj.com/articles/china-stalls-global-search-for-coronavirus-origins-wuhan-markets-investigation-11589300842.

Patrick S. (2020), *When the System Fails*, "Foreign Affairs", 99(4).

Poast P. (2020), *Competitors, Adversaries, or Enemies? Unpacking the Sino-American Relationship*, *War On The Rocks*. Available at: https://warontherocks.com/2020/10/competitors-adversaries-or-enemies-unpacking-the-sino-american-relationship/.

Prideaux J. (2020), *Checks and Balance: How China might save the West*. "The Economist".

Reinhart C., Reinhart V. (2020), *The Pandemic Depression: The Global Economy Will Never Be the Same*, "Foreign Affairs", 99(5).

Runde D. F., Savoy C. M., McKeown S. (2020), *Covid-19 Has Consequences for U.S. Foreign Aid and Global Leadership*, *Center for Strategic and International Studies*.

Available at: https://www.csis.org/analysis/covid-19-has-consequences-us-for-eign-aid-and-global-leadership (Accessed: 9 February 2021).

Schrader M. (2020), *Analyzing China's Coronavirus Propaganda Messaging in Europe*, *GMF Alliance for Securing Democracies*. Available at: https://securingdemocra-cy.gmfus.org/analyzing-chinas-coronavirus-propaganda-messaging-in-europe/ (Accessed: 9 February 2021).

Silver L., Devlin K., Huang C. (2020), *Unfavorable Views of China Reach Historic Highs in Many Countries*. Available at: https://www.pewresearch.org/global/2020/10/06/unfavorable-views-of-china-reach-historic-highs-in-many-countries/.

The Economist (2020), *Hurly-barley*, 26 November. Available at: https://www.econ-omist.com/asia/2020/11/26/could-australias-government-have-handled-china-better.

The Economist (2021), *Covid-10trn*, 9 January. Available at: https://www.econo-mist.com/finance-and-economics/2021/01/09/what-is-the-economic-cost-of-covid-19.

Uehara M., Tanaka A. (2020), *China to overtake US economy by 2028–29 in COVID's wake: JCER*, "Nikkei Asia", 10 December. Available at: https://asia.nikkei.com/Economy/China-to-overtake-US-economy-by-2028–29-in-COVID-s-wake-JC-ER.

United States Strategic Approach to The People's Republic of China (2020). Available at: https://www.whitehouse.gov/articles/united-states-strategic-approach-to-the-peoples-republic-of-china/.

Wisniewski R. (2019), *Chinese vision of international order – implications for Central Asia*, in: Wallas T., Stelmach A., Wiśniewski R., *Beyond Europe Reconnecting Eurasia*. Berlin: Logos.

Wisniewski R. (2020), *Wpływ współpracy i rywalizacji mocarstw na bezpieczeństwo międzynarodowe w Azji Północno-Wschodniej w latach 1989–2014*. Poznan: Wydawnictwo Naukowe Wydziału Nauk Politycznych i Dziennikarstwa UAM.

Radosław Fiedler
Adam Mickiewicz University, Poznan
ORCID 0000-0003-1573-9898

WHY DID THE US FAIL TO RESPOND TO COVID-19?[1]

The COVID-19 pandemic caused by a novel coronavirus – Severe Acute Respiratory Syndrome Coronavirus 2 (SARS-CoV-2) – surprised the majority of states and severely strained the health system capacity. In the beginning, in Wuhan, China, several weeks later – spread globally. In response, governments decided to halt all social and economic activity to slow down the spread of highly infectious coronavirus and prevent paralysis of the entire health system. The COVID-19 pandemic and looming health crisis, and even collapse coerced governments to act decisively at the expense of the economy. In the first quarter of 2020, the Eurozone economies shrank at a 14.8 % annualized rate and in the US, nearly 28 million persons filed new claims for unemployment benefits over the six weeks ending April. The coronavirus crisis has been characterized as a "reallocation shock" due to the freezing of sectors of professional activity requiring personal contact– mainly tourism, airlines, hospitality, food services, health care, and entertainment – have been subject to a specific shock and may remain depressed for a long time (Barrero, Bloom, Davis 2020).

Considering the high social and economic costs, not to mention the ongoing health crisis raises the question: why did previous coronavirus outbreaks not affected so severely globally? SARS-CoV-2 is not the first health crisis in the twenty-first century connected to a coronavirus. In 2003, the outbreak of Severe Acute Respiratory Syndrome Coronavirus 1 (SARS-CoV-1) was the first global call for an emergency. Eventually, the outbreak was stopped, the animal sources were eliminated from the markets, and in-

---

[1] The research was financed from the project „Research on COVID-19" from the funds of the Adam Mickiewicz University, Poznan.

fected people were isolated. Their number reached 8,098 cases. Altogether, SARS claimed 44 lives in Canada out of a total of 438 probable cases. Globally, estimated mortality was relatively low 916 but a pretty terrifying mortality rate —11 percent of those infected. The World Bank has estimated that the SARS epidemic caused an estimated $54 billion in worldwide economic loss. However, the biggest part of this sum was not constituted by direct care costs, but, as Michael T. Osterholm and Mark Olshaker highlighted, it was the effect of "aversion behavior" on the part of the public (Osterholm, Olshaker 2017, 139). Nine years later, in 2012, another life-threatening coronavirus appeared, namely, Middle East Respiratory Syndrome: Coronavirus (MERS CoV). The infectious centre was located in Arabian Peninsula. Fortunately, it did not expand globally. In that example, the virus was transmitted from dromedaries, a type of camel. Even though camel owners' did not kill their valuable and culturally important animals. Fortunately, MERS stayed only regional health crisis. There are more than 1.2 million dromedary camels in the Arabian Peninsula, and 78 percent of them are found in Saudi Arabia, the United Arab Emirates, and Yemen (Osterholm, Olshaker 2017, 141). Presently, it can not be excluded that a more infectious variant of the MERS may spread much more easily and globally. Fortunately, in those earlier cases, the most effective measures against the spreading of the virus lay in limits of SARS and MERS, which infected only certain individuals as superspreaders. It was unpredictable just who those superspreaders would be and, unlike COVID-19, which can be transmitted by unaware carriers, SARS and MERS usually become highly infectious until the fifth or sixth day of symptomatic illness (Osterholm, Olshaker 2020).

SARS-CoV-2 pandemic has entered the second year and will be a global challenge in the coming years. Different and more contagious variants came several waves and enforced governments to impose lockdowns. Israel, United Kingdom, and the United States are leading in vaccination efforts to decrease the spreading of the virus and to considerably lower the mortality rates. Other countries are also are following the suit. Vaccination and immunity would mean a return to normalcy without social distance and potential V-shaped economic recovery. Despite that optimistic perspective seemed to be within the grasp, uncertainty remains that the new coronavirus variant may be more resilient to the vaccine, which, in the coming months, could result in concurrently imposing lockdowns and short-lived openings in many countries. Recurring lockdowns caused by new variants of coronavirus are preventing economic recovery and deepening the health crisis.

The impact of the COVID-19 global pandemic is difficult to assess because of its multiple regional and global effects. We need to consider its negative impact on individuals, whole societies, education, disruptions of social direct interactions of individuals, children, and youth, economy, trade, tourism, entrainment, culture, gastronomy, and intensifying tensions in international politics. The pandemic also revealed the problem of strained global supply chains. Disruptions in global supply chains that are being observed amid COVID-19 are not new phenomena. Earlier were natural disasters caused temporary disruptions in needed parts In the past, the IT industry was severely affected by floods in Thailand, which wiped out a large proportion of global hard drive capacity, and by the Fukushima earthquake which also had a considerable impact on electronic and chemical supply chains. In March and April of 2020, the COVID-19 pandemic caused shock on the global supply chains and its long-lasting effects and fragility of globalized networks have initiated changes. The situation is redefining the rules behind globalization. Nowadays, slow globalization marked by regionalization is often considered as a remedy for building resilience against the shortage of critical demand products. The coronavirus pandemic has left some of the world's biggest shipping lines facing mounting backlogs and delays, straining international supply chains and threatening to disrupt global trade COVID-19 have placed particular pressure on the availability of containers which directly has raised the cost of transporting containers more than 100% since March 2000 (Stephens 2021).

Strained global supply chains are also coinciding with the rise of US-China tensions. The US's idea that China's growing integration with the global economy would additionally liberalize its political system turned out to be naïve. Globalized supply chains provided resources for certain repressive governments or, in the case of China, helped in providing a rationale for the ruling party to continue its dominance and a greater global influence and multiple leverages in negotiations with the US (Mensah 2010: 13).

In addition to the slowdown and partial freezing of economies in individual countries, the pandemic has severely hit entire sectors globally, including the airline-industrial complex. In 2019 4.5bn passengers were air passengers. Over 100,000 commercial flights a day have filled the skies. The global airline sector was supported by 10 million employees directly not including additional services as TAXI, Caffe, meals, language handlers, 2.7m airline workers; and 1.2m people in building and repairing planes. Altogether they helped generate revenues of $170bn for the world's airports and $838bn for airlines (Economist, 1 August 2020)

The airline-industrial complex may recover, however, a much more complicated problem is related to more than 1.5bn students around the world who have been forced out of classrooms and seen their education has been disrupted by the Covid-led closure of schools and colleges (Fearn, 2021). Based on observations, one can assume that COVID-19 has strengthened more powerful and centralized governments, and big technological and pharmaceutical companies have gained much more data on individuals and whole societies, which were additionally supplied by contact-tracing technologies and vaccination.

The process of digitalization, Artificial Intelligence (AI), automatization and robotization, and the possibility of remote work had been known before the pandemic. The COVID-19 has accelerated and developed those trends and probably in one pandemic year has been done progress accentuated for several years. The current wave was shaped by the invention of the microprocessor almost fifty years ago and concurrently came the revolution in the new information and Communication Technologies (ICTs) such as the internet and robotics, Big Data, and AI (Nübler, 2020: 192).

The question is why the United States, one of the richest countries in the world, was so severely affected by the COVID-19 epidemic with many negative consequences and a death toll of 600,000?

In the macroeconomic data presented by Joseph Stiglitz, GDP growth in the US was positive from 1947 to 1980, the US grew at an annual rate of 3.7 percent, while for the last third of a century, from 1980 to 2017, the average growth rate has been only 2.7 percent, a full percentage point lower (Stiglitz 2018:47). This is not only a problem of slowing down the dynamics of GDP growth but also of increasing income differences and social injustice in American society. Robert Reich writes a lot about the failing American economic model. According to him, tens of millions of Americans live in poverty. As Reich emphasizes, "almost 30 million Americans still lack health insurance, most workers who lose their job aren't eligible for unemployment insurance, one out of five American children lives in poverty, and nearly 51 million households can't afford basic monthly expenses such as housing, food, child care, and transportation. Our infrastructure is crumbling, our classrooms are overcrowded, and our teachers are paid far less than workers in the private sector with comparable levels of education" (Reich 2020: 37). America has become famous around the world as the country that has put more people in prison (relative to its population) than any other country. Amazingly, the United States has 25% of the world's prisoners, though it has but 5% of the world's population, and these prisoners are disproportionately African American (Stiglitz 2018: 190).

In the book The Great Reversal, Thomas Philippon lists the shortcomings of the American system in which big corporations have a privileged position. He has noticed that in the US they have been allowed to report a huge proportion of their foreign profits in small, low-tax jurisdictions. Such opportunities and many other ones in various areas are not just being exploited. They are being actively created, through lobbying (Philippon 2019: 153–156).

Other indicators of inequality in the US are unequal access to healthcare and insufficient welfare care. What has exposed the US the most, is its lagging behind in terms of the availability of hospital beds per 1,000 inhabitants compared to other highly industrialized countries. Japan has 13 beds per 1,000 people, while the US has fewer than three beds per 1,000. And this is just one statistical variable. There are large national differences in key inputs such as ICU beds, ventilators, hospital protective equipment, and healthcare workers (Philippon 2019: 223–239).

Another indicator is the low life expectancy in the US, although between 1959 and 2016, the US life expectancy increased from 69.9 years to 78.9 years, it has declined for 3 consecutive years after 2014. The recent decrease in the US life expectancy culminated in a period of increasing cause-specific mortality among adults aged 25 to 64 years that began in the 1990s. The reasons for this situation are associated with improper diet, lack of exercise, drug overdoses, alcohol abuse, suicides (Woolf, Schoomaker 2019).

The above-mentioned factors created favourable conditions for the fact that the first wave of COVID-19 took such a heavy toll from the beginning. Although The spring 2020 surge generated deaths largely in New York, parts of New England, Louisiana, and Georgia, the fall 2020 surge is widespread nationally, with hot spots in rural states and on both coasts. Notably, people of colour have about twice the death rate as White people; 1 in 875 Black persons and 1 in 925 Indigenous persons have died compared with 1 in 1625 White persons. Other high-risk groups for Covid-19 infection include essential workers, prisoners, and prison staff (Koh, Geller, Tyler 2021).

As in other countries affected by the COVID-19 pandemic, seniors are the group with the highest mortality. Compared with those aged between 18 and 29 years, people between the ages of 75 and 84 years and those aged 85 years or older have 200 times and 630 times greater average death rates, respectively (Centers for Disease Control and Prevention 2020). Nursing homes and long-term care facility residents and staff are at high risk, representing only 5% of the population but 38% of deaths. In 14 states, at least half of deaths have been linked to nursing homes; in 6 states, the percentage is more than 60%, in 3, 70% or more (New York Times, 4 December 2020).

Since the first case of COVID-19 in the US was confirmed on January 20, it took almost two months for the federal government to acknowledge the risk of COVID-19 and implement decisive measures. Despite the increasing number of infections, President Trump downplayed the threat of the disease in January and February, in many public statements, especially on Twitter, President Trump assured that the COVID-19 epidemic did not threaten the US and that each case was under control. One such example was his tweet from February 24, 2020, which read: "The Coronavirus is very much under control in the USA. We are in contact with everyone and all relevant countries. CDC & World Health have been working hard and very smart. Stock Market starting to look very good to me!" (Trump Twitter Archive 2020).

While analyzing Trump's statements, one could get the impression that the president did not realize what challenge he would have to face. Nothing could be more inaccurate, President Trump had been warned by his advisers on January 28, 2020. Just on this day at the top-secret intelligence briefing, a senior official has informed President Trump that coronavirus will be the "biggest national security threat" of his presidency. (Woodward 2020: 181). More importantly, while the Trump administration took office in January 2017 there were, among other things, plans to produce cheaper ventilators and 20 million reusable face masks, should the country need them but failed to continue that path. In 2018 John Bolton, the national-security adviser, changed the National Security Council and closed its pandemic preparedness office. The following year, the administration decided to no longer embed an epidemiologist from the Centres for Disease Control and Prevention (CDC). (Economist 11 April 2020).

Although the federal authorities took several counteractions, they proved to be overdue and not enough to mitigate the impact of the first wave of COVID-19.

Measures that were undertaken to mitigate the surge of infections of COVID-19 in January 2020:

- On January 17, the Centers for Disease Control and Prevention (CDC) announced that 3 airports in the US would begin screening incoming passengers from China: SFO, JFK, and LAX Other 2 airports were added subsequently, and on January 28, the U.S. Department of Health and Human Services (HHS) announced that 15 additional U.S. airports (bringing the total to 20) would begin screening incoming travelers from China.

– On Jan. 31, the U.S. Centers for Disease Control and Prevention (CDC) issued a federal quarantine for 14 days affecting the 195 American evacuees from Wuhan, China. Starting Sunday, Feb. 2, U.S. citizens, permanent residents, and immediate family who have visited China's Hubei province will undergo a mandatory 14 days quarantine and, if they have visited other parts of China, they would be screened at airports and asked to self-quarantine for 14 days. The last time the CDC had issued a quarantine was over 50 years ago in the 1960s, for smallpox.

– The White House was considering issuing a ban on flights between the United States and China, as of late Jan. 28. Italy has announced on January 31 that it was suspending all flights to and from China (Goodman, Schulkin, 2020). March 11, 2020: The World Health Organization (WHO) declares that COVID-19 is a global health pandemic. That same day: President Trump announces new travel restrictions from 26 European countries. Initial travel restrictions did not apply to the United Kingdom.

It was not possible to reduce the tide of infections and the rapidly increasing number of deaths proved that the situation was very difficult. In both the US and South Korea, the first confirmed case of COVID-19 was traced on January 21, 2020. South Korea launched an extensive program to counteract COVID-19 and within five weeks sixty-five thousand were tested while the US reached only five hundred (Seulki, Jungwon, Chongmin 2020: 243–260). Not only the delayed response but also the inconsistency in countering Covid-19 and most importantly throughout the election year - politicization. Dr Francis Collins, the director for the National Institutes of Health (NIH), emphasized in one of the interviews that particularly president Trump and other Republicans who dismissed mask-wearing during the coronavirus pandemic could cost tens of thousands of lives (Mastrangelo 2021). An illustration of such a situation was President Trump's reluctance to cooperate with experts should also be mentioned (Kirlin 2020: 467–479). President Trump's supporters from the very beginning demanded that he dismiss dr. Anthony Fauci, director of the National Institute of Allergy and Infectious Disease. In response to their expectations, the president minimized the participation of experts in press conferences.

Besides, the complex US federal structure is also a challenge in successfully countering the COVID-19 pandemic. In 57 jurisdictions (50 states, 5 territorial health departments, New York City, and the District of Columbia). For example, in the US's federal system the timing of shelter-in-place orders and other population-wide measures aimed at stopping the spread of the virus and similarly, the decision of ending lockdown were under the responsibility of cities and states (Economist 30 May 2020). As noted by Xuefei: "Collaboration among different levels of the government has been fatally inadequate. Those states with the highest numbers of infections, such as New York and New Jersey, have been urging the federal government to redistribute urgent supplies such as ventilators and N95 masks. Without centralized redistribution, states must compete with one another while bidding for critical medical supplies in the private market" (Xuefei 2020: 430).

In the early May of 2020, an American was dying of COVID-19 every forty-nine seconds. The US, with 4% of the world's population, had more than 30 percent of the sick (Sternfeld, Egan 2020: 12). Andrew Cuomo, the governor of New York, despite being criticized for not introducing pandemic restrictions earlier, gave the feeling, both to the residents of the state but also all Americans, that only the systemic approach could be counteracted against the pandemic. As he observed, COVID-19 has exposed many shortcomings and came while American society is deeply divided and polarized. He enlisted eight critical points that should be adapted to a more efficient response to the pandemic crisis as follows: 1. There should be clearly defined lines of responsibilities and authority between the various levels of government during a health crisis; 2. An early detection system of domestic and international public health threats is essential; 3. The leadership of public health organizations tasked to respond to future public health threats must be able to operate free from political interference; 4. The government's response to public health threats must be informed and guided by data; 5. The federal government must build a public health emergency operation team and program with the capacity to coordinate and respond to major health crises; 6. The country must have a health screening system as part of its border patrol control system; 7. State governments must reinvent the public health capacity, 8. Citizen action is needed and responsible observance of all the rules to contain infectious diseases (Cuomo 2020, 221).

Cuomo had to deal with a tremendous wave of the pandemic. New York has become a hot spot. Paramedics and hospitals lacked protective gear, not to mention the insufficient number of ventilators. On March, 29, New York reported 965 deaths and 59,513 confirmed cases, accounting for more than 40% of America's cases and 7% of the world's. The majority of these—678 deaths and 33,768 cases were in New York City (Economist 29 March 2020).

On one hand, the growing number of victims of the pandemic, and on the other, the deteriorating condition of the economy and the threat of permanently increasing unemployment, forced the Trump administration, and above all the Republicans and Democrats, to work out a program of financial aid beyond political divisions and as soon as possible. At the end of March 2020, a 2 trillion dollar stimulus bill – the CARES Act – passed both the House of Representatives and the Senate and was signed by President Trump. The bill provided a one-time payment of a $1,200 check for individuals making up to $75,000 per year or $2,400 for couples earning less than $150,000. It also includes loans to businesses, funds unemployment insurance, bails out airlines and cargo carriers, authorizes aid to states and defers taxes, and other financial aid (Timeline of the Coronavirus Pandemic and U.S. Response 2020).

The huge financial aid program helped to avoid a more serious crisis or even a recession, but it did not improve President Trump's political ratings. Even before the lockdown, in February 2020, the president was almost guaranteed a second term. In times of crisis, societies usually tend to unite with their leaders despite political divisions. 9/11 was such an example, the Americans rallied around President George W. Bush who initially had bad ratings. However Trump was unable to utilize this capital, and he was merely addressing his electorate, divided instead of unifying, and was judged negatively for his chaotic response to COVID-19.

In Joe Biden's presidential campaign, getting out of the pandemic was a key task, only after that, it was possible to move on to the next stages, such as sustained economic growth. In a 20-minute address delivered in a conversational tone, he called on Americans to come together to tackle the pandemic and economic downturn during what he described as a "winter of peril and significant possibilities".

A month after President Joseph Biden's inauguration, the COVID-19 surge continued to cause a health crisis. February 22, was marked by 500,000 official deaths. The pandemic caused more deaths than the first world war, second world war, and Vietnam war, combined (Economist 17 March 2021).

A priority for Biden's administration has been a massive vaccination campaign, and more importantly, 200 million Americans were successfully vaccinated in the first 100 days of his presidency.

Conclusions

The initial response by the US government to COVID-19 was marked by a lack of recognition of the risk that the infectious disease had posed. Since the first case was confirmed in mid of January, it took almost two months for the federal government to acknowledge the risk of COVID-19 and implement decisive measures. Despite the increasing number of infections, President Trump has downplayed the threat of the disease in January and February, stating that the coronavirus is under control. However, it is too simplistic to blame the Donald Trump administration for the high death toll as well as tens of millions of COVID-19 infections. Beyond failures of the federal government, one should also add failures of local and state government in delayed response to the COVID-19 pandemic. Ironically, in some respects, COVID-19 may have been a stabilizing force. In the US, the pandemic may have helped bring an end to the presidency of Donald Trump. Had Trump been reelected the rollback of American democracy, rule of law, domestic political division and declining American would have accelerated.

However, the problem is much more complicated and touches the essence of the social and economic model around which the American society has been organized. The article enumerates the following problems and limitations that have been inherited by Biden's administration: a weak health and social protection system, lower life expectancy caused also by the wrong diet, high level of inequality, racial injustice, and absence of public provision of health care. Full availability is required of employees, but adequate social protection is not guaranteed. Overcoming the pandemic does not rely only on a mass vaccination program, but also on the reconstruction of the existing socio-economic model, which is a task for many years. A strongly polarized society poses a serious problem and political conflicts can prevent major changes in an ailing system.

It is worth noting The American Rescue Plan Act, the economic stimulus bill in US history prepared by Joe Biden's administration. The program includes $1,400 one-off cheques for Americans earning up to $75,000 a year, an extension of federal unemployment benefits, and thousands of dollars in tax credits for children, among other provisions (Fedor 2021). Moreover, the Biden administration is preparing a program of large infrastructure investments with the possibility of modernizing outdated infrastructure and stimulating employment and economic growth.

A much more difficult task will be the reconstruction of the social system, and above all, enabling unlimited access to health care. The COVID-19 pandemic will probably last long enough to initiate needed changes. Despite the serious political divisions in the US, the financial aid program enjoys support regardless of political preferences. Will it be possible to create a bipartisan consensus to fix failures? The Rescue Financial bill is a step in the right direction and economic recovery indicators are visible. In 2020, the US experienced a health disaster, but in 2021 it has become a world leader again in the mass vaccination program and a gigantic financial program also addressed to those most in need of support and prospects for the V-shaped recovery. This gives hope for a renewal of the American Dream.

References

Air travel's sudden collapse will reshape a trillion-dollar industry (2020), https://www.economist.com/business/2020/08/01/air-travels-sudden-collapse-will-reshape-a-trillion-dollar-industry (Accessed: March 10, 2021).

Scrikbayeva B., Abdulla K., Oskenbayev Y. (2020), *State Capacity in Responding to COVID-19*, "International Journal of Public Administration".

Barrero J., Bloom M., Davis S. (2020), *COVID-19 Is Also a Reallocation Shock*, "Brookings Papers on Economic Activity", Summer 2020.

Bigger than Trump. The White House v covid-19Now that the Trump administration has taken charge of the government's pandemic response, how is it doing? (2020), https://www.economist.com/united-states/2020/04/11/the-white-house-v-covid-19, (Accessed: March 10, 2021).

Cohen S. (2021), *Looking Back and Looking Ahead After a Year of Pandemic* https://blogs.ei.columbia.edu/2021/03/08/looking-back-looking-ahead-year-pandemic, (Accessed: March 10, 2021).

COVID-19 hospitalization and death by age. (2020), Centers for Disease Control and Prevention https://www.cdc.gov/coronavirus/2019-ncov/covid-data/investigations-discovery/hospitalization-death-by-age.html, (Accessed: March 10, 2021).

Coumo A. (2020), *American Crisis. Leadership Lessons from the COVID-19 Pandemic*, Random House LLC, New York.

Cutler D. M., Summers L. H. (2020), *The COVID-19 Pandemic and the $16 Trillion Virus*, "JAMA", https://jamanetwork.com/journals/jama/fullarticle/2771764, (Accessed: March 10, 2021).

Koh H.K, Geller A. C., VanderWeele T. J. (2020), *Deaths From COVID-19* (2020), "JAMA", https://jamanetwork.com/journals/jama/fullarticle/2774464, (Accessed: March 10, 2021).

Fearn N.(2020), *Remote learning shows the power of the cloud to transform education. Post-pandemic, colleges will have the potential to extend the reach of quality teaching;* "Financial Times", https://www.ft.com/content/3596847e-a981-42c0-8a6c-bc1c52d5cf04, (Accessed: March 10, 2021).

Fedor L. (2021), *Popularity of US stimulus puts Republicans in a bind*, "Financial Times", https://www.ft.com/content/aff82e56–4fcf-4098-bf75-adb71aa8ecf1, (Accessed: March 10, 2021).

Blendon R. J., Benson J. M., Schneider E. C. (2020), *The Future of Health Policy in a Partisan United StatesInsights From Public Opinion Polls* (2021), "JAMA", https://jamanetwork.com/journals/jama/article-abstract/2777394, (Accessed: March 10, 2021).

Mensah S. (ed.) (2010), *Globalized supply chains and U.S. policy*, Nova Science Publishers, New York.

Goodman R., Schulkin D. (2020), *Timeline of the Coronavirus Pandemic and the U.S. Response*, https://www.justsecurity.org/69650/timeline-of-the-coronavirus-pandemic-and-u-s-response/ (Accessed: March 10, 2021).

Horwitz J. (2020), *Facebook to Shift Permanently toward More Remote Work after Coronavirus*, "Wall Street Journal", 21 May 2020.

Kirlin J. (2020), *COVID-19 Upends Pandemic Plan,* "The American Review of Public Administration". 2020;50(6–7):467–479.

Morath E., Lang H. (2021), *February Hiring Sets Up Stronger Spring Recovery. Restaurant employment booms amid renewed consumer spending and fewer restrictions,* "Wall Street Journal" https://www.wsj.com/articles/february-jobs-report-unemployment-rate-2021–11614909553, (Accessed: March 10, 2021).

Murray Ch. J. L., Piot P. (2020), *The Potential Future of the COVID-19 Pandemic Will SARS-CoV-2 Become a Recurrent Seasonal Infection?* "JAMA", https://jamanetwork.com/journals/jama/fullarticle/2777343?resultClick=1, (Accessed: March 10, 2021).

New York Times (2020), *Nearly One-Third of U.S. Coronavirus Deaths Are Linked to Nursing Homes* Published December 4, https://www.nytimes.com/interactive/2020/us/coronavirus-nursing-homes.html, (Accessed: March 10, 2021).

Nübler I. (2020), *Shaping the Work of the Future: Policy Implications*, in: *Work in the Future The Automation Revolution*, Skidelsky R.,Nan C. (eds,), Palgrave Macmillan.

Mastrangelo D. (2021), *NIH director: Mask politicalization may have cost 'tens of thousands' of lives in US*, https://thehill.com/homenews/administration/539820-nih-director-mask-politicalization-may-have-cost-tens-of-thousands-of, (Accessed: March 10, 2021).

Osterholm M. T., Olshaker M. (2017), *Deadliest enemy. Our war against killer germs*, Little Brown and Company, New York

Osterholm M. T., Olshaker M. (2020) *Learning From the COVID-19 Failure—Before the Next Outbreak Arrives*, "Foreign Affairs", https://www.foreignaffairs.com/articles/united-states/2020-05-21/coronavirus-chronicle-pandemic-foretold, (Accessed: March 10, 2021).

New York is fast becoming the world's next coronavirus hotspot (2020), "The Economist", https://www.economist.com/united-states/2020/03/29/new-york-is-fast-becoming-the-worlds-next-coronavirus-hotspot, (Accessed: March 10, 2021).

Philippon T. (2019), *The Great Reversal How America Gave Up on Free Market*, The Belknap Press of Harvard University Press, London

Reich R. (2020), *The System. Who Rigged It, How We Fix It*, Alfred A. Knopf, New York.

Seulki L., Jungwon Y., Chongmin N. (2020), *Learning before and during the COVID-19 outbreak: a comparative analysis of crisis learning in South Korea and the US*, "International Review of Public Administration", 25:4, (Accessed: March 10, 2021).

Stephens P. (2020), *Supply chain 'sovereignty' will undo globalisation's gains. The search for national 'resilience' can too easily tip into protectionism*, "Financial Times", https://www.ft.com/content/b5f72f88-814f-4697-8b83-e7d120c81fdc (Accessed: March 10, 2021).

Sternfeld J., Egan T. (2020), *Uprepared. America in Time of the Coronavirus*, Bloomsbury Publishing, New York.

Stiglitz J. (2018), *People, Power, and Profits Progressive Capitalism for an Age of Discontent*, W.W.Norton and Company, London New York, New York 2017.

Trump Twitter Archive (2020), https://www.thetrumparchive.com/?results=1&searchbox=%22coronavirus%22, (Accessed: March 10, 2021).

Woolf S. H., Schoomaker H. (2019), *Life expectancy and mortality rates in the United States, 1959–2017.* "JAMA". 2019;322(20):1996–2016, (Accessed: March 10, 2021).

Woodward Bob (2020), *Rage*, Simon&Schuster, New York.

Xuefei R. (2020) *Pandemic and lockdown: a territorial approach to COVID-19 in China, Italy and the United States*, Eurasian Geography and Economics, 61:4–5.

Beata Bochorodycz
Adam Mickiewicz University, Poznań
ORCID: 0000-0002-9415-8129

JAPAN'S RESPONSE TO COVID-19. TOWARDS STRATEGIC AND NONSTRATEGIC COOPERATION[1]

Japan's response to the coronavirus pandemic is difficult to assess clearly in early 2021 when the third wave is passing through the Japanese archipelago. Prime Minister Suga Yoshihide, who in September 2020 took over the post after the longest-serving prime minister in the history of Japanese parliamentarism, Abe Shinzō, declared a second state of emergency on January 8 and then 12, 2021, for several most populous prefectures. Nevertheless, by the end of 2020, with fewer infections, a lower number of deaths, a lower rate of deaths, and without strict lockdowns, Japan, compared to the United States and Europe, seemed effective in fighting the pandemic. In addition to the domestic arena, Japan, deeply embedded in various international and regional institutions, was particularly active and responsive to a variety of initiatives by such organizations as the World Health Organization (WHO) or the International Monetary Fund (IMF). What contributed to this apparent success? What were the policy decisions and their underlying causes made by national actors in response to the COVID-19 crisis? What were the effects of those policies on Japan's position in the global system? The article tackles these questions paying special attention to the patterns of cooperation and competition between Japan and various international actors on domestic, regional, and global levels.

---

[1] I am deeply indebted to Sigur Center for Asian Studies at George Washington University in Washington for access to the library resources. My special thanks go to prof. Mike Mochizuki and prof. Benjamin Hopkins, the director of the Center. The research was financed from the project „Research on COVID-19" from the funds of the Adam Mickiewicz University, Poznan.

The article argues that although the impact of COVID-19 on Japan's public health and economy has been severe, it has not fundamentally changed Japanese health, security, or economic policies, but rather accelerated earlier trends caused by the growing power of China and hegemonic rivalry with the United States as well as other market-driven forces. Furthermore, the article suggests that although severe competition and total decoupling from China is not an option for Japan, which has strongly promoted the cooperative engagement with its giant neighbor, in the post-COVID-19 world Japan is most likely to clearly distinguish between strategic and non-strategic cooperation and deepen the strategic cooperation for securing the critical supply chains with its allies and like-minded partners under the Free and Open Indo-Pacific (FOIP), Quadrilateral Security Dialogue (QUAD) and other frameworks.

Note that the article covers the period of 2020, that is Japan's first wave of April-May, and the second wave of July-August, while the third wave, which began in November 2020 and was incommensurately larger in scale and number, is largely omitted, although the general conclusions apply to it as well. The article is divided into three sections, of which the first part discusses Japan's domestic policies in response to the pandemic, the second part analyzes the regional initiatives of Japan's government, and the third part examines the global engagement of Japan aimed at the containment and mitigation of the COVID-19 impact.

Domestic Response

Japan's success of the first waves

By the end of 2020, Japan seemed to handle the pandemic relatively well despite a high population density (in Tokyo twice higher than in New York) and the large percentage of high-risk individuals over 65 years old (over 25%). The data gives convincing evidence for this success. From the beginning of the pandemic in January 2020 until the end of 2020, Japan recorded 233,725 cases of COVID-19 including 3,459 deaths (MHWL, 2021b), which was below 0.3% of all deaths in 2020 (Kōsei Rōdōshō, 2020a)[1]. By comparison, six times more people died from suicide, which number has been in decline for a decade (Keisatsuchō, 2021). In terms of deaths per million people (DPM) as of January 20, 2021, that is, during the third wave of the pandemic, Japan performed much better than Europe or the United States. By comparison to other Asian countries, such as China – 3.34, Mongolia – 0.61, South Korea – 25.67, and Taiwan – 0.29 DPM, Japan with 37.79 DPM had the highest mortality. Nevertheless, in the global context, with the world average 266.17 DPM (as of 20 Jan. 2021), and the worst-performing countries in Europe, such as Belgium – 1775.04, Italy – 1384.03, U.K. – 1376.85, Spain – 1158.59, France – 1099.86, Poland – 902.09, Germany – 596.89, all hard-lockdown countries, not to mention the USA – 1227.02 DPM, Japan scored relatively much better (Our World in Data, 2021).

At the same time, it turned out that Japan managed to achieve such a result without draconian restrictions. According to the Oxford University **Government Response Stringency Index**, which measures the strictness of nine lockdown measures including school closures; workplace closures; cancellation of public events; restrictions on public gatherings; closure of public transport; stay-at-home requirements; public information campaigns; restrictions on internal movements; and international travel controls – Japan stayed under 50 out of 100 points (the strictest). During the April state of emergency, Japan's highest point was 47,22, while by comparison, other developed economies during the same time reached the following stringency levels: Italy – 93.52, France – 87.96, Poland – 83.33, UK – 79.63, USA – 72.69, Sweden – 64.81, with only Taiwan keeping far below with 31.48 points (data for 21 April 2020; Hale at al., 2020).

There are several reasons behind Japan's apparent success in coping with the first waves. According to Omi Shigeru and Oshitani Hitoshi, two members of the government advisory panel on COVID-19, five main factors contributed to Japan's success in mitigating the first wave with a relatively small number of infections and deaths (Omi and Oshitani, 2020: 2). First, easy access to medical care under the national health insurance system, which covers practically all Japanese, foreign permanent residents, and long-term visitors; second, generally high quality of medical care and easy access, even in rural areas, with hospitals supported by a national network of local public health centers (*hokenjo*); third, the Japanese public's high standard of hygiene, willingness to comply with government requests, and other cultural traits and lifestyle habits; fourth, early detection of transmission waves and prompt introduction of countermeasures; and fifth, the cluster-based approach (Omi and Oshitani, 2020: 2). While the first three factors have been indicated by other sources and publicized by mass media, the last two were added by the experts based on their work for the government in various expert committees. Both Oshitani and Omi are recognized international experts on infectious diseases who have held many important posts and led WHO global initiatives. The third cultural factor, as usually, is debatable and often employed when other explanations do not suffice, although intuitively, it seems reasonable to assume that a society with high hygiene standards, habits of frequent washing of hands and mouths, wearing masks, usually keeping distance in face-to-face interactions, and other habits, is less prone to spread of contagious diseases. In the context of such cultural habits, some of the WTO initiatives, such as the #WearAMask campaign, which was met with protests in some countries (e.g., USA, Germany, Poland) and treated as an infringement on civic freedoms, in Japan did not require any special actions because wearing a mask is already deeply embedded in the public health culture, as well as in other Asian countries. The seasonal outbreak of cold, flu or even pollen season is met with a high rate of voluntarily mask-wearing, not to spread the virus and to protect oneself. This has been sometimes mistakenly perceived by Europeans and Americans as a sign of protection against heavy air pollution. In addition to the above success factors, I would also mention the government's deep involvement and the broad scope of countermeasures that were introduced in fighting the pandemic. Interestingly, the Japanese public has been much less appreciative of governmental efforts than international experts and organizations, a theme I will return to later on.

Government's institutional response

Japan's government's institutional response to the first outbreak at the beginning of 2020 seemed relatively swift. On January 30, 2020, the same day WHO declared the global emergency, Japan government established in the Cabinet Secretariat that is directly under the Prime Minister command, a **Novel Coronavirus Response Headquarter** (hereafter as Response HQ) by the Cabinet Decision (see Table 1). Japan as a centralized system of government, constitutionally guarantees a high degree of local autonomy to prefectures and basic units of local government (*shichōson*), but both legally and customarily, the central government is expected to take the lead and coordinate activities for tackling major social, political and economic problems, not to mention emergency situations such as pandemics. The degree of citizens' expectations towards the central government reflects the structure of the political system but also of political culture. In Japan, both expectations and demands on the central government have been very high, and so the public criticism. The Response HQ was therefore to coordinate national efforts with local governments, which established similar headquarters in each prefecture, and other state institutions, as well as to enhance the cooperation with international institutions in fighting the pandemic. The Response HQ was headed by the Prime Minister and vice-chaired by Chief Cabinet Secretary, the right-hand man of prime minister, the Minister of Health, Welfare and Labour (MHWL), and the newly designated State Minister for Special Measures Law for Novel Influenza. Other members include all state ministers and a secretary, that is a bureaucratic official designated by the prime minister. In addition, there is also a secretariat (*kanjikai*) composed of bureaucratic representatives of all ministries and governmental offices relevant to the issue of the pandemic, at least forty people in total. On March 26, the Response Headquarter was given the status of Government Response Headquarter (hereafter Government Response HQ), which put it under the Special Measures Law for Novel Coronavirus, thereby strengthening its legal base.

Under the Response HQ (and later Government HQ), **Novel Coronavirus Expert Meeting** (hereafter Expert Meeting), was set on February 14, 2020, which operated until July 3, 2020. The aim of the Expert Meeting was to assist the government with specialistic knowledge on public health, and consisted of ten experts from those areas, chaired by Wakita Takaji, the president of the National Institute of Infectious Diseases (NIID), and vice-chaired by above-mentioned Omi Shigeru, the president of the Japan Community Healthcare Organization (JCHO). As mentioned, Omi is a leading figure in Japan in the area of public health and contagious diseases and served at WHO engaging in global health initiatives. The chairperson Wakita is a physician and a researcher specializing in contagious diseases. The role of the experts was very substantial during the first waves of the pandemic and strongly affected policy measures.

To strengthen the legal basis of governmental bodies and their activities, on March 13, 2020, Japan's parliament enacted legislation that enabled the government to declare a state of emergency over the coronavirus outbreak. It was actually a revision of a law adopted in April 2012 in response to the outbreak of another infectious disease, the influenza H1N1 pandemic in 2009 and outbreaks of other flues (e.g., the bird flu). For that reason, it was named **Special Measures Law for Novel Influenza** (Shingata Infurenza to

Taisaku Tokubetsu Sochihō), and since March 2020, after the revision, the law has been known otherwise as Special Measures Law for Novel Coronavirus (hereafter SML for Coronavirus, Shingata Coronauirusu Tokusohō).

Table 1. Institutional arrangements for tackling the pandemic

Response HQ (Novel Coronavirus Response Headquarter; Shingata Koronauirusu Kansen Taisaku Honbu) ▼ (changed to) Government Response HQ (Government Response Headquarter; Seifu Taisaku Honbu)	Expert Meeting (Novel Coronavirus Expert Meeting; Shingata Koronauirusu Kansen Taisaku Senmonka Kaigi)		
	Ministerial Meeting (Ministerial Meeting on Measures Against Avian Influenza; Shingata Infuruenza tō Taisaku Kakuryou Kaigi)	Advisory Council (Advisory Council on Countermeasures against Novel Influenza and Other Diseases; Shingata Infuruenza tō Taisaku Yūshikisha Kaigi)	Basic Action Policy Advisory Committee (KihontekiTaishoHōshintōShimonIinkai)
			Expert Subcommittee (Subcommittee on Novel Coronavirus Disease Control; Shingata Koronauirusu Kansenbyō Taisaku Bunkakai)
	Ministry of Health, Welfare and Labour (MHWL)	MHWL Advisory Board (Novel Coronavirus Advisory Board; Shingata Koronauirusu Kansenbyō Taisaku Adobaizarii Bōdo)	Various working groups

S o u r c e: Compiled by the author.

On April 7, 2020, the government announced the state of emergency based on the recommendations of the **Basic Action Policy Advisory Committee,** chaired by Omi Shigeru. The Advisory Committee, the statutory body under the SML for Novel Coronavirus, was conveyed on March 27 by the Government Response HQ to advise on the situation. The Advisory Committee comprises all ten members of the Expert Meeting and eight other specialists in the fields of medicine and public health. Once the state of emergency was announced, other statutory bodies were conveyed. The **Basic Action Policy Advisory Committee** formally is placed under the jurisdiction of **the Advisory Council on Countermeasures against Novel In-**

fluenza and Other Diseases (hereafter Advisory Council), which again is under **Ministerial Meeting on Measures Against Avian Influenza** (hereafter Ministerial Meeting). The Advisory Council is the largest assembly of non-governmental specialists that advise the government, comprising over thirty members, including all Expert Meeting members, from predominantly public health and medical circles, in addition to business and labor organizations, media, local government, and others. It is also chaired by Omi Shigeru and vice-chaired by Okabe Nobuhiko. Okabe, from Kawasaki City Health and Safety Research Institute, is another leading specialist of infectious diseases with experience of working at WHO. The Ministerial Meeting, composed of state ministers, was originally established by oral consent (so not as a Cabinet Decision) in September 2011 to coordinate governmental efforts by the Cabinet ministers to tackle the outbreak of the novel influenza. During the 2020 coronavirus pandemic, it was conveyed for the first time on April 12, 2020, after the state of emergency was declared on April 7, 2020.

When the first wave retreated, the **Novel Coronavirus Expert Meeting** was dissolved in July 2020, and a new body of the **Subcommittee on Novel Coronavirus Disease Control** (hereafter Expert Subcommittee) was established on July 3, 2020, under the Ministerial Meeting, and more specifically under its **Advisory Council on Countermeasures against Novel Influenza and Other Diseases**. It was in fact an expert team composed of twenty members, including all ten members of the former Expert Meeting. The main difference between the Expert Meeting and the new Expert Subcommittee was that in the former body almost all members were experts and specialists from public health and medical institutions (except one layer), while in the latter there were specialists from other areas of business and labor organizations, and local governments. In addition, legally, a new subcommittee was established within the framework of the SML for Coronavirus. The subcommittee was chaired by Omi Shigeru, who served also as the vice-chairperson of the Expert Meeting. It was this subcommittee that on January 5, 2021, advised the government on the second state of emergency, which Prime Minister Suga declared on January 8, 2021.

Another expert committee under the name of **Novel Coronavirus Advisory Board (hereafter MHWL Advisory Board)** was conveyed on February 7, 2020, by the MHWL, which was composed of all members of the Expert Meeting (est. Feb. 14), and chaired by Wakita Takaji (Kōsei Rōdōshō, 2020–2021). After the second meeting on February 10, the committee was not conveyed until July 14, 2020, that is after the Expert Meeting was dissolved and Expert Subcommittee established. The purpose of the Advisory Board was to exchange "free and open opinions" and advise the MHWL, as expressed by the MHWL Minister Katō Katsunobu during the July 14 meeting (Kōsei Rōdōshō 2020b: 2). This committee included strictly public health-related specialists.

To sum it up, the committees of experts specializing in the fields of medicine and public health were analyzing the data and advising the Japanese government under the framework of Government Response HQ between February and July 2020 and since July 2012 under the Ministry of Health, Welfare and Labour, first as Expert Meeting and then as Advisory Board. The core of the public health specialists in all expert bodies was composed of the same people, which allows for a smooth flow of information. At the same time, since July 2020, the committee of specialists under the Government Response HQ, the Expert Subcommittee was expanded to include representatives of other fields such as business, labor, local government, and media. Normatively, the institutional change was to streamline the organizational structure of the government's pandemic command. However, symbolically, it can also represent a shift from a strictly science-based approach to a broader interests inclusive-approach in tackling the crisis. The success in containing the first waves of the pandemic was achieved with a great economic cost, and so during the later stages, the government tried to minimize the economic impact, postponing decisions and restrictions as long as possible until the situation became very serious. Furthermore, institutionally, the approach to the pandemic has been to create specific normative frameworks (e.g., SML for Novel Influenza in 2012) that have to be revised and adjusted whenever a new situation occurs, and thus not as a permanent feature of the system.

Restrictions of the First Wave

Japan's restrictions in comparison to other countries, as disused above and indicated by Government Response Stringency Index, were relatively mild. The decisions were made both with the advice of the expert committees in response to the unfolding domestic situation and in response to global developments and calls from international organizations.

The first coronavirus infection in Japan was confirmed on January 16, 2020, in a resident of Kanagawa Prefecture who returned from Wuhan, that is, seven days after Chinese state-run media reported on the detection of the first novel coronavirus in a patient. On January 28, the first patient in Japan, who had not traveled abroad, was confirmed. The border restrictions followed quickly. On February 1, the authorities banned entry for travelers from Hubei province and to all Chinese passport holders, which was expanded to travelers from Zhejiang province on February 12. Second, on March 27 travelers from Italy, Germany, France, and other parts of Europe were denied entry, and then on April 3 from the United States, Britain, and the rest of China. For other non-travel restrictions, it took almost a month before the government introduced certain measures. On February 26, large-scale gatherings were suspended, and the following day on February 27, Prime Minister Abe requested schools to close. All in the form of recommendations without penalty. On March 24, the government announced the postponement of the 2020 Tokyo Olympic and Paralympic Games to 2021. One of the widely publicized developments of that time was the entry of the cruise ship Diamond Princess to Japan and placing it under quarantine in Yokohama port on February 3 after the group infection was confirmed among passengers and crew members. In total, more than 700 of the 3,711 people on board got infected and 13 died (Kōsei Rōdōshō, 2020c).

On April 7, Prime Minister Shinzō Abe declared a state of emergency for Tokyo, and six other prefectures (Kanagawa, Chiba, Saitama, Osaka, Hyogo, and Fukuoka) to prevent further spread of infection. The state of emergency was expanded nationwide on April 16 and lasted until May 6. The government called for extensive business closures to a wide range of local businesses and private facilities, including public universities and schools, athletic facilities, live houses, concert halls, and community centers, as well as bars, nightclubs, net cafes, and other nightlife destinations. During the press conference on April 7, Prime Minister Abe famously stated that "In order to move on from the state of emergency in one month, we must reduce people-to-people contact by 70%, ideally by 80%," calling on citizens to cooperate (Cabinet Secretariat, 2020). Interestingly, there were no penalties for noncompliance, which differed from the second state of emergency. Nevertheless, the Japanese citizens and companies seemed to follow the request, refraining from going out and shortening business hours. According to the data of NTT DoCoMo's mobile phone operator, one of the largest in Japan, the number of people around Shibuya Station in Tokyo, a famous shopping and entertainment district, decreased by 65% during weekdays and 77% during holidays as analyzed by the location of mobile phones between April 13–19 in comparison to the preceding months of January and February 2020

(Asahi Shinbun, 15 Jan. 2021, p. 16). More importantly, by the beginning of May, the total number of infected persons fell gain under 100 per day, with total deaths well under 500 (MHWL, 2021a).

Cluster-based approach

Japanese public health experts advising the government recommended several measures, such as washing hands, wearing masks, social distancing, all of which were strongly suggested by WHO (e.g., WHO's *Interim Guidance* of 10 January 2020) and other institutions, but in addition, a cluster-based approach to tackle the pandemic at an early stage. Analyzing the data available as of the end of February 2020, the experts concluded that over 80% of infected people in Japan did not transmit the virus to others and that most of the transmissions occurred via clusters (group infections) (Oshitani and Omi, 2020). With the total infection number in the country low, the remedy was to trace back the activities of infected people, to identify the ways of transmission (retrospective tracing), and at the same time to educate the public and prevent future cluster formations (prospective tracing). Furthermore, the analysis of the common environmental and behavioral characteristics allowed to identify three settings that foster the occurrence of clusters, labeled as Three Cs, discussed below. The cluster-based approach was fully implemented during the first wave from February to April 2020 (Oshitani and Omi, 2020; Oshitani et. al., 2020). The experts estimated that to flat the curve and stop the transmission, close contact would have to be reduced by 80% (Oshitani et. al, 2020: 491), and this is the figure that Prime Minister Abe mentioned during the declaration of the first state of emergency. At the end of March 2020, the number of unidentified epidemiologic links increased, which meant that more chains of transmissions were not identified. Because the identification was conducted via interviews with infected persons, it meant that some people were not willing to disclose information about their activities (e.g., visiting nightclubs and bars). The state of emergency, which introduced this cluster-based approach, began reaching its limits later due to the increased number of infections and difficulty in monitoring all cases, and thereby the growing strain on the health system. The surge in infection as indicated by the virus effective reproduction number, that is, the number of people that one infected person infects stayed under one during the first state of emergency (Oshitani and Omi, 2020: 8). The problem would grow more serious at the end of 2020 during the third wave, but during the first wave of the pandemic in April-May, the cluster-based approach seemed to work, and the situation was brought under control.

Concerning the cluster-based approach, the Japanese government relied on a few strategies that were skillfully framed and propagated, such as, for instance, "the three Cs" (*Mitsu no Mitsu*), "Three Cs Plus", or "Five Situations". The concept of the "three Cs" (Photo 1), which is basically a social distancing measure, denotes high-risk places and situations that most often contribute to transmissions and outbreaks of infectious diseases, such as (1) Closed spaces with poor ventilation, (2) Crowded places with many people nearby, and (3) Close-contact setting such as close-range conversations. The risk of occurrence of cluster infections was assumed to be high when the "three Cs" overlapped, and so the public was asked to avoid them. The Three Cs Plus expanded the above by including such behaviors as laud talking and singing (Three Cs Plus) (Oshitani and Omi, 2020: 7). The last item means that the popular entertaining facilities of karaoke are to be avoided. Finally, the ways of propagating the virus countermeasures (washing hands, 3Cs, clusters, decreasing contact by 80%, etc.) were seemingly effective as catchy phrases were repeated and reprinted widely by state and private media, posters, and audio announcements in public spaces.

Social stigmatization

One of the social phenomena that draw public and media attention was the stigmatization of the sick but also of the medical staff. Already in April 2020, the Expert Meeting prepared a report, in which such cases were described. The experts listed prejudice and discrimination against medical and welfare employees of medical institutions and welfare facilities for the elderly, where large-scale infection cases have occurred; against people engaged in occupations that are essential for maintaining social functions such as logistics; or even against children of the above-mentioned professions or other infected people, who were refused entry to kindergarten or school (Kantei, 2020c: 6). At one point, some celebrities were even making public "apologies" for being infected with the coronavirus. The experts warned that such situations not only make the life of patients and their families difficult but also raise the risk of infection spread because people might delay reporting, which again might delay the detection of infections. Furthermore, as experts argued, stigmatization and prejudice might lower the motivation of health and welfare employees, encourage leave and turnover, which ultimately might lead to the collapse of the medical system in Japan. The government and the media began a campaign for rising awareness and eradicating discrimination and prejudice, although the problem has remained.

Domestic Economic Measures

Dealing with the economic consequences of the pandemic, the Japanese government, like many others around the world, was striving for a balance between public health and the health of the economy. The government's requests for refraining from going out, for social distancing, shortening business hours, shifting to home, office, and others, were followed by support measures for businesses and individuals. On February 13, the government announced the **1st COVID-19 emergency response package**, which included home return support for Japanese travelers abroad, and loan support for small and medium enterprises (SMEs). On March 10, the government announced **the 2nd COVID-19 emergency response package**, with such key measures as additional loan support for companies and strengthening employment support measures. On April 7 (amended April 20), the government proposed **the 3rd emerging economic package** to stimulate the economy. The total scale of the package was 117 trillion yen (USD 1.1 trillion), equivalent to 20 percent of the country's GDP. About seventy-five percent of the budget was allocated to employment and business support, and the rest to healthcare systems, consumption promotion campaigns, and public investment, etc. The package titled: **Emergency Economic Measures in Response to COVID-19** to protect the lives and lifestyles of the public and move toward economic recovery in support of business included, first, real interest-free unsecured loans, improved loan conditions allowing recurring debts to be refinanced as interest-free loans, deferment of the payments of national taxes and social security premiums without collateral and penalties (amounting to JPY 26 trillion); second, cash payments (app. JPY 15 trillion), including cash payments of 100,000 yen to all residents of Japan, including nonresident foreigners such as exchange students (JPY 12.9 trillion), and cash payments of 2 million yen each to micro-, small-, and medium-sized business and 1 million yen each to individual business owners (JPY 2.3 trillion in total); third, demand stimulation measures for the period after the containment of outbreaks, such as discounts and vouchers for individuals to be used for commodities and services in such sectors as tourism, transport, food services, and event businesses (Kantei, 2020b). On May 27, the government announced an **additional economic stimulus package** of the total package of 117 trillion yen (same as the 3rd emergency economic package) with key measures of rent fee support benefits for SMEs and subordinated loans for large companies. Finally, on June 12, an **extra budget** of a record 31.91 trillion yen (USD 309 billion) was enacted to mitigate social and economic fallout from the coronavirus pandemic. Altogether, the government secured the COVID-19 contingency fund of 5 trillion yen in the FY2020 budget and promised another 5 million yen in the FY2021 budget to contain the pandemic, mitigate its impact and prepare for future infection outbreaks (MOF, 2021).

Together with the domestic economic measures, Japan also committed substantial resources to IMF and World Bank to assist low-income developing countries, as I will discuss later. For both actions, Japan was hailed by IMF Managing Director, Kristalina Georgieva as an example to follow for the sizable economic and fiscal measures "to alleviate the health challenges and support households and business to bridge through the economic challenges" (IMF, 2020). Despite governmental economic measures, the real gross domestic product (GDP) for the April-June period as compared to the previous quarter decreased by 29.2%, which was the worst record since the end of the war in 1945 (*Asahi Shinbun*, 15 Jan. 2021, p. 16). This is one of the reasons that when the third wave of infections began around November, the government was reluctant to declare a state of emergency again and waited till the beginning of January 2021. The government's position became a target of criticism. One of the controversies involved the initiative "Go-To-Travel", aimed at boosting the domestic tourism and service industry. On December 11, 2020, the same day when Omi Shigeru, the chairperson of the Expert Subcommittee, announced the necessity to stop the campaign due to a rapidly increasing number of infections, Prime Minister Suga during a TV program maintained that the government had no intention of canceling the initiative (*Asahi Shinbun*, 25 Dec. 2020, p. 18). Finally, on January 28, 2021 PM Suga finally announced the suspension of the program, but the issue is also representative of the deep sociopolitical and economic tensions brought up by the health crisis. The government was trying to promote economic policy while keeping an eye on the pandemic situation, balancing public health and the health of the economy.

Politics of Public Opinion

Despite relative success in tackling the pandemic, the general public in Japan has been rather critical of the government's actions. The approval rate of the government for tackling the coronavirus has been fluctuating but generally, the number of people dissatisfied with the countermeasures grew over the period between April 2020 and January 2021 (see Table 2). The NHK, the national broadcasting station, has been conducting the poll monthly. In April 2020, 46% of Japanese replied that they positively evaluated the government's efforts, while the majority of 50% were negative (NHK, 2020a). In July, after suppressing the first wave, the public grew a little more approving, with 50% positively evaluating the government and 45% negatively (NHK, 2020b). However, that was the only time when the majority positively viewed the government's efforts. In December 2020, 41% evaluated the government positively and 56% negatively (NHK, 2020c). The percentage of dissatisfied voices grew again larger in January 2021, raising to 58%, while the number of satisfied people dropped to 38% (NHK, 2021). Although this type of satisfaction is highly subjective and thus not reflecting the actual situation or relative success of Japan in comparison to other states, it is although indicative of certain perceptions and expectations of citizens towards its government (both politicians and bureaucratic officials).

Table 2: Satisfaction with the government's response to COVID-19

	April 2020	July 2020	Dec. 2020	Jan. 2021
Positive (positive + very positive)	46% (8% + 38%)	50% (5% + 45%)	41% (4% + 37%)	38% (3% + 35%)
Negative (negative + very negative)	50% (36% + 14%)	45% (35% + 10%)	56% (40% + 16%)	58% (41% + 14%)

S o u r c e: Based on NHK, 2020a, 2020b, 2020c, and 2021.

The so-called public opinion politics has become an important feature of the Japanese political landscape since Prime Minister Koizumi Jun'ichirō (2001–2006), who skillfully used traditional and new media, including social media, to balance the power of his own party factions and carry out public policies. Since then, consecutive cabinets have been sensitive to public sentiment as expressed in opinion polls, conducted by a variety of public (e.g., NHK, Cabinet Office) and private institutions (e.g., all major dailies).

The audience cost for the Cabinet is thus high, and so the economic and financial measures to help the micro, small and medium-size enterprises, self-employed, individual households, or big corporations in securing jobs are as much a result of rational economic planning as of electoral calculations, alike the situation in most liberal democracies.

Strategic and nonstrategic supplies

Medical supplies

The outbreak of the pandemic disrupted Japan's supply chains, because, like many countries around the world, Japan has relied on overseas production, mostly in China. "Supply chains" became a buzzword denoting various commodities depending on the stage of the pandemic. Generally, the government designated some supplies as strategic with regard, first, to medical and public health commodities, and second, to other products essential for national security and interests. The division of supplies into strategic and nonstrategic had practical consequences for business operations. The production of strategic supplies was to shift back to Japan (reshoring) or to the countries considered as Japan's allies or partners under such arrangements as, for instance, Free and Open Indo-Pacific (FOIP) or QUAD (Quadrilateral Security Dialogue) (nearshoring).

One of the first concerns for the government at the outset of the pandemic was clearly to secure the provision of medical and health commodities. Japanese authorities resorted to a policy of special measures to encourage domestic production. The government-private sector cooperation has a long tradition, as was famously introduced by Charmers Johnson and labeled as "developmental state" in his acclaimed book, *MITI and the Japanese Miracle* (Johnson, 1982). MITI or the Ministry of International Trade and Industry was the predecessor of METI (Ministry of Economy, Trade and Industry since 2001), which together with the Ministry of Health, Welfare and Labour (MHWL) were at the forefront of negotiations with the private sector both domestically and globally. The first main governmental agency that traditionally oversees foreign relations was the Ministry of Foreign Affairs (MOFA). The extent of government leadership in tackling the pandemic, and of cooperation, involvement in the economy and business was very extensive and congruent with previous practices.

Already in February 2020, before WHO's call of March 3, for "for industry and governments to increase manufacturing by 40 percent to meet the rising global demand in response to the shortage of personal protective equipment endangering health workers worldwide", the government of Japan announced **FY2019 Subsidy Project for Supporting Businesses in Introducing Facilities for Producing Face Masks** (WHO, 2021). On February 28, METI nominated three companies (Kowa, XINS, Hata Industries) to be provided with subsidies for installing production equipment by the second week of March, while on March 13, METI designated eight more enterprises (Allegro-Knit, Consortium of Sharp Corporation, Shirohato, Hokuriku Web. etc.) to support domestic production (METI, 2020d). On April 15, 2020, a week after the declaration of the state of emergency, the government organized the first **Meeting with Companies Contributing to the Increased Production of Personal Protective Equipment and Other Supplies**. During the meeting, Prime Minister Abe thanked the business community for cooperation and declared that "we must firmly secure the production of such important supplies, which are crucial to public health and their supply chain in Japan. With such a sense of urgency, we have decided to implement bold budgetary measures by increasing the subsidy rate for capital investment to encourage business operators" (METI, 2020e). The domestic production was to include surgical masks, sanitizers, and personal protective equipment such as medical gowns, medical devices including ventilators, and the antiviral drug Avigan, which seemed effective in aiding the treatment of patients with COVID-19 (*The Japan Times,* 17 Dec. 2020). Prime Minister Abe announced that the government secured for that purpose 250 billion yen at that time (METI, 2020e). The governmental special measures aimed at encouraging domestic production included subsidies for capital investment to mask factories and other manufacturing facilities, support for the procurement of raw materials, expediting the screening process for the approval of new ventilators, and deregulation on alcohol use. The authorities also gave a guarantee to purchase all remaining and unsold supplies for national reserves. In the following months, METI announced several programs to this end, in May – FY2020 Subsidy Project for Supporting Businesses in Introducing Facilities for Producing Protective Clothing (Kezai Sangyōshō, 2020a), and FY 2020 Subsidy Project for Supporting Businesses in Introducing Facilities for Producing Ventilators and Other Medical Equipment (Kezai Sangyōshō, 2020b), and in July – Program for Promoting Investment in Japan to Strengthen Supply Chains (METI, 2020f). For the last program, METI selected 146 projects amounting to about 247.8 billion yen in total (METI, 2020f), which included both (a) products, parts, and materials largely produced overseas (56 projects), such as semiconductor parts or materials, aircraft parts, electric vehicle battery parts or materials, rare metals, and displays, and (b) products, parts, and materials essential for people's wellbeing (90 projects), such as antiseptic alcohol, masks and surgical masks (including parts), medical gowns, and medical gloves. Altogether, 299 firms complied with the governmental request and on December 2, 2020, METI Minister Kajiyama Hiroshi granted certificates of gratitude to companies and associations "for their great contributions to stabilizing people's daily lives amid the pandemic of the novel coronavirus disease for their urgent increase in the production of medical supplies in response to METI's requests and other calls to improve demand and supply." At the commendation ceremony held in the METI building, the Minister handed the certificates of appreciation to few representatives of those firms (METI, 2020c).

In the meantime, to stabilize the supply of face masks and contain the buying spur, on March 15, the government **prohibited the resale of face masks**, in accordance with the Act on Emergency Measures for Stabilizing Living Conditions of the Public. Furthermore. In preventing the practice of bulk buying and reselling facial masks at inflated prices, or on auction sales, METI secured cooperation from such giant platforms as Yahoo!, Japan and Mobaoku. Furthermore, the Ministry also encouraged companies to sell their unnecessary stockpiles to relevant markets at reasonable prices (Kantei, 2020a). With the increased production and import, the government announced that it was able to secure a supply of over 600 million face masks in March (METI, 2020e). In addition to the procurement, the government attempted to stabilize the distribution by establishing a national system for the preferential supply of medical goods to medical facilities nationwide in cooperation with Japan Medical Association and the Japan Dental Association, two influential interest, and advocacy organizations. The government requested that relevant associations of manufacturers and wholesalers preferentially supply 410,000 surgical masks to 14 municipalities, and 188,000 surgical masks to 68 designated medical facilities for infectious diseases (METI, 2020e).

Initially, the shortage of face masks and other medical goods led to a short consumer panic facilitated by SNS and other media informing about a shortage of toilet paper and facial tissues, among others. The METI and Japan Household Paper Industry Association had to issue special statements, assuring that the production lines and distribution of these products were in normal operation. They also explained in detail the supply chain, namely, that forty percent of the pulpwood, which is the raw material of these products manufactured in Japan, is imported from North and South America, and not from China or other Asian countries. METI posted on its site the following appeal: "METI asks consumers to act calmly and rationally and not to buy these products for reselling them or stocking up on them beyond normal use amounts. These actions may hinder the distribution of these products to those who need them. Thank you for your understanding and cooperation" (METI, 2020e). The majority of the Japanese most probably accepted the explanation because the buying spur ended quickly.

Nevertheless, the fact that authorities, companies, and other organizations had to ensure the public that certain products, parts, or raw materials do not come from China is very illustrative and symptomatic. Since the mid-1980s, the Plaza Agreement, and the devaluation of the Japanese yen, Japan has largely shifted its production base overseas not only in the case of medical and health products. In fact, over 50% of Japanese manufacturing takes place overseas, largely in China, ASEAN, the US, and Europe (David, 2020). In addition, among the industrialized and developed countries, Japan has the lowest rate of self-sufficiency of food, which is not directly related to the pandemic in terms of health, but it raises general concerns about disruption of supply chains (Nōrin Suisanshō, 2019). The public fear that the pandemic might disrupt the supply chains was thus legitimate. Japan's prompt response to the crisis in the case of medical and health supplies stemmed rather from its production structure and supply chains, and therefore the acute awareness of the urgency of the situation.

Regional cooperation

Chine Plus One

The division into strategic and nonstrategic commodities, securing and diversifying their supply chains has begun long before the present pandemic, but the COVID-19 undeniably accelerated Japan's attempt at restructuring its supply chains (Nagy, 2021). Both regarding strategic and nonstrategic supplies, the Japanese companies started shifting their production sites out of China much earlier, following the China Plus One supply chain management strategy. There were several factors contributing to this shift such as China's uncertain growth outlook over the last decade, increasing costs (e.g., procurement and labor costs), earlier experiences with supply disruptions during the Koizumi and Noda cabinets as a result of anti-Japanese sentiments and overseas public protests,[2] and finally, the impact of the most recent U.S.-China trade war including the confrontation over the cutting-edge technologies. The "trend out of China" was confirmed by the Teikoku Databank survey of June 2019, which showed a decline in the number of Japanese companies in China from a peak of 14,394 in 2012 to 13,934 in 2016, and 13,685 at the end of May 2019 (*NNA Business News,* 3 June 2019). Another poll conducted by Nikkei showed that 23.9% of Japanese companies indicated that they are preparing to change their international supply network already in 2019 (Nakafuji, 2019). The COVID-19 pandemic did not thus start but has accelerated this trend. In February 2020, 37% out of 2,600 companies that responded to a survey conducted by Tokyo Shoko Research Ltd, answered that they were planning to diversify their procurement to places other than China (David, 2020).

For the strategic and nonstrategic supplies, there have been generally three main directions of expansion of the production network for Japanese companies, first, Southeast Asia, especially ASEAN and more recently, India and Bangladesh, and second, other close allies and partners, such as Australia, and third, back to Japan, as partially discussed above. It is worth noting that the directions of nearshoring are congruent with the political and security strategies of the Japanese government envisioned under the Free and Open Indo-Pacific (FOIP) or Quadrilateral Security Dialog (QUAD). The third direction, reshoring that is back to Japan, is also linked to the Japanese government policy of enhancing domestic industrial security of strategic commodities to ensure the provision of critically important goods for Japan's domestic market also in areas other than public health. Those products are to be made at home to prevent exposure to trade disruptions due to rising geopolitical and other risks in the region. One of those designated as critically important (strategic) goods for national security, along with medical and public health products (since COVID-19), pharmaceuticals, and telecommunications, has been semiconductors. METI allocated 110 billion yen in the fiscal 2019 budget and an additional 90 billion yen to an extra budget to boost manufacturing advanced chips domestically. In January 2021, the media reported that the chip giant Taiwan Semiconductor Manufacturing

Company (TSMC) would build an advanced packaging facility in Japan in cooperation with METI, which has been lobbying for this investment for some time (*The Japan Times*, 6 Jan. 2021).

The first direction of expansion for Japanese companies to Southeast Asia, especially to ASEAN countries, has been under way for over a decade due to relatively low labor and power costs, openness to foreign investment, and young population. Despite the history of Japanese militarism, according to the survey by Singapore-based ISEAS-Yusof Ishak Institute, Japan is considered the most trusted major power among the Southeast Asian nations, in fact, the only one that is trusted by the majority, 61.2% (Tang et al., 2020: 49). Japanese investment into the region rose at almost double the pace of China from 2011–2012, including Vietnam, Thailand, Indonesia, Malaysia, and the Philippines (Takeo and Jamrisko, 2020). In June 2020, Japan External Trade Organization (JETRO), an agency closely related to METI, announced the first 30 companies to receive state subsidies worth 12 billion yen (USD 114 million) under the **Program for Strengthening Overseas Supply Chains** to expand their production base to ASEAN countries. The program supported by the ASEAN Economic Minister-METI Economic and Industrial Cooperation Committee (AMEICC) is to strengthen "supply chain resilience including support for the construction of additional manufacturing plants and enhancement of production/logistical efficiency by utilizing digital technologies" (JETRO, 2020). The aim is to reduce the reliance of Japan on China or any other individual state as a manufacturing source. By September that year, the subsidy program that reached by that time 23.5 billion yen (USD 221 million) in the 2020 supplement budget, was to be extended to India and Bangladesh (*Nikkei*, 4 Sept. 2020, p. 4).

The first and second direction of expansion (other allies and partners) for Japanese business has been India and Australia, in line with the Free and Open Indo-Pacific concept. Both countries have been increasingly important partners for Japan not only under the FOIP framework. Australia has been in fact the second, after the United States, a military ally since 2007. As the COVID-19 pandemic progressed, METI in cooperation with India and Australia lunched the **Resilient Supply Chain Initiative** (RSCI) announced in September 2020 to deliver "a free, fair, inclusive, non-discriminatory, transparent, predictable trade and investment environment" (METI, 2020b). Amitendu Palit from the Institute of South Asian Studies in the National University of Singapore was quick to declare in an article printed in an influential journal, The *Diplomat*, that RSCI was "one of the first examples of a distinct anti-China geoeconomic alliance taking shape in the post-COV-ID-19 world", and furthermore, that it "symbolizes segregation of global and regional supply chains along geopolitical lines" with "the wider possibility of the post-COVID-19 global economic order being fashioned into distinct blocs of cross-border production networks representing specific political alliances" (Palit, 2020). Repositioning strategic supply chains of semiconductors, pharmaceuticals, and telecommunications from China to countries without security threats is clearly a sign of geostrategic considerations, but is it really a sign of an effort to "decouple from China in a broader strategic sense"? It's rather doubtful. China has been Japan's biggest economic partner since 2006. In the near future, China will most probably become the biggest economy in the world in terms of GDP. Although some Japanese companies, as shown above, are planning to leave China to diversify their production network, the majority (over 60%), and especially those producing commodities destined for Chinese markets, are determined to stay (Nakafuji, 2019; David, 2020). The apparent economic decoupling, if it can be called decoupling at all, is occurring only partially in the sphere of strategic supply chains. The nonstrategic products and those produced for the Chinese vast market are most likely to stay in place. As noted by several scholars focusing on Japan (Nagy, 2020a, 2020b; Hosoya, 2019; Soeya, 2020), Japan as a middle power has pursuit cooperative engagement rather than competition or containment of China, while using cooperation and collaboration among like-minded partners "to ensure the region's evolution includes their interests" (Nagy, 2020b: 3).

Other Regional Initiatives

While securing strategic supply chains, Japan has been engaging in multilateral frameworks of economic and political cooperation to ensure access for Japanese companies to markets across the Indo-Pacific and beyond. Regarding China, Japan has been consistently trying to balance and engage its powerful neighbor. China Plus One supply chain management strategy aimed at diversification of production networks, which does not mean total decoupling, but rather restructuring those relations or, in other words, "selective decoupling" (Nagy, 2021).

Since the early stage of the pandemic, Japan has kept in touch with regional partners and institutions. Already on April 14, 2020, the **Special ASEAN Plus Three (Japan, China, and ROK) Summit on Coronavirus Disease**

2019 (COVID-19) was held via a video conference, which was also attended by the WHO Director-General in addition to regular members. Prime Minister Abe referred to regional preventive measures against the spread of the virus, including sharing information and knowledge "freely, transparently, and timely", but also proposed the establishment of an ASEAN Centre for Emerging Diseases and Public Health emergencies (tentative) as a way to prevent future crisis (MOFA, 2020e). Another event, the Special ASEAN Plus Three Economic Ministers' Virtual Conference Meeting on COVID-19 Response took place on June 4, after which the ministers issued *ASEAN Plus Three Economic Ministers' Joint Statement on Mitigating the Economic Impact of the COVID-19 Pandemic.* The joint statement, except references to the pandemic, touched upon various other issues such as "keeping the markets open to strengthen the resiliency and sustainability of regional supply chains", or refraining from "taking unnecessary measures that may affect the smooth flow of essential goods such as medicines" (METI, 2020a). The ministries also emphasized the commitment to signing the **Regional Comprehensive Economic Partnership (RCEP)** agreement. And indeed, RCEP has been one of the most ambitious projects at engaging China and building a regional cooperation framework, although not as comprehensive as the Comprehensive and Progressive Agreement for Trans-Pacific Partnership (known otherwise as TPP11). The pandemic did not stop those efforts and finally on November 15, 2020, Japan together with China, Australia, and 12 other countries (most notably without the US) signed the agreement, creating thereby the world's largest trading bloc, accounting approximately for 30% of the global GDP. India has not joined the agreement in the end, but the doors have been left wide open. The agreement was in fact a joint initiative of Japan and China introduced at the East Asia Summit Economic Ministers in 2011. The pandemic indeed disrupted negotiations at the beginning of 2020, but the talks were resumed via videoconferences, and at least nine of them included the highest-level officials. Other regional events, such as, for instance, East Asia Summit was also held online in November 2020 and hosted by Vietnam, where the summit was initially scheduled to occur (ASEAN, 2020). To complicate the above picture and show the complexity of regional relations, it is worth noting that few days after signing the RCEP on November 15, 2020, Japan and Australia signed a defense pact, which allows the partners to share bases during military exercises and disaster missions. Prime Minister Suga together with Australia's Prime Minister Scott Morrison in a Joint Statement "affirmed that trade should never be used as a tool to apply political pressure" because it undermines trust and prosperity (MOFA, 2020b: 5). While engaging its powerful neighbor, Japan together with its allies and partners are hedging against China (Nagy, 2021).

Global cooperation

On the global level, Japan's response to COVID-19 challenges was in many ways exemplary, as hailed by the aforementioned IMF Managing Director, Kristalina Georgieva (IMF, 2020). Since the end of the Cold War, while maintaining strong relations with its main ally, the United States, Japan has pursuit multilateralism and international collective action not only in the economic sphere but also in global and regional security, playing a more significant leadership role than has been usually recognized (Midford, 2020). Such multilateralism does not preclude bilateral or trilateral agreements. The coronavirus pandemic thus provided Japan with a chance to further enhance its international position, and actively partake in global initiatives. In comparison to the United States under the Trump administration, Japan has been a strong advocate of international organizations, voicing its support for UN (MOFA, 2020a), WHO (MOFA, 2020b), and for other organizations such as IMF or World Bank (Aso, 2020).

Japan engaged in IMF's initiatives, such as the **Catastrophe Containment and Relief Trust** (CCRT) and the **Poverty Reduction and Growth Trust** (PRGT). First, CCRT is to provide grants for the relief of IMF debt services for the poorest and most vulnerable states, which were hit hard this time by the coronavirus, while second, PRGT is to provide emergency financing for developing countries to meet their imminent needs to combat COVID-19. As the largest contributor to IMF financial resources, and concessional lending facilities, Japan has provided close to SDR 9 billion (23% of all PRGT loans) and over SDR 0.9 billion in subsidy grant resources (close to 15% of total contributions) (IMF, 2020). In response to calls by IMF, World Bank Group, and other International Financial Institutions for urgent contributions to address critical funding needs, on April 8, 2020, Japan pledged a contribution of an additional 100 million USD to the CCRT as immediately available resources to IMF, and on April 16, its intention to double its contribution to the PRGT from the current SDR 3.6 billion, making the first SDR 1.8 billion available immediately (IMF, 2020). Japan called also on other member states to join the initiative.

Universal Health Coverage, COVAX AMC, and Gavi

Japan has played a prominent role in advancing the global health agenda, especially since the G8 Okinawa Summit in 2000, hosted by Japan, during which the issue of infectious disease control was extensively discussed, and the initiative of the Global Fund was launched. Japan has also been spearheading a number of innovative health initiatives such as a loan conversion mechanism for its long-standing polio eradication program support and promoting Universal Health Coverage (UHC) as the overarching approach for attaining Sustainable Development Goals (SDG3). In December 2018, Japan proposed the establishment of a Group of Friends of UHC with the purpose to serve as an informal platform for UN member states to coordinate efforts towards establishing UHC by 2030, as stated in the Political Declaration of the High-level Meeting on Universal Health Coverage, as well as in the Sustainable Development Goals. The Group consists of 64 member countries and areas, and as of 2020, it was co-chaired by Thailand, Georgia, and Japan.

The platform of Group of Friends of UHC was used during the pandemic to respond to the COVID-19 crisis. On October 8, 2020, Japan co-hosted a virtual Ministerial Meeting of the Group of Friends of Universal Health Coverage (UHC), chaired by Minister for Foreign Affairs, Motegi Toshimitsu. It was attended by Secretary-General of the United Nations – António Guterres, Director-General of WHO – Tedros Adhanom, the Coalition for Epidemic Preparedness Innovations, foreign ministers or other officials representing Thailand, Georgia, Kenya, Senegal, Ghana, Uruguay, India, UK, France, EU, and other representatives from the private sector and civil society. Under the slogan of "leaving no one's health behind" and based on the principle of human security, Foreign Minister Motegi outlined the three pillars of Japan's initiative (MOFA, 2020d). It included 1) developing countries' capacity to tackle COVID-19, including equitable access to vaccines under the COVAX AMC framework, 2) strengthening health systems in preparation for future health crises, and 3) generating an enabling environment for health security.

COVAX AMC or the COVID-19 Vaccines Advance Market Commitment was launched at that Global Vaccine Summit earlier that year on June 4, by Gavi, the Coalition for Epidemic Preparedness Innovations (CEPI), and WHO. As an innovative financing instrument, the aim is to guarantee fair and equitable access for every country in the world, especially to 92 low- and middle-income economies to safe and effective COVID-19 vaccines (Gavi, 2020a). At the Global Vaccine Summit in June 2020, Japan pledged 130 million USD for COVAX AMC (approx. 6.5% of all donors) to ensure equitable access to COVID-19 vaccines (Gavi, 2020b). It was part of the total of 300 million USD that Japan committed to providing to Gavi for 2021–2025.

Gavi, previously known as the GAVI Alliance, and before that as the Global Alliance for Vaccines and Immunization, was one of the initiators of the COVAX AMC project. Gavi, a public-private global health initiative to increase access to immunization to poor countries, was originally set up in 2000 when the Bill & Melinda Gates Foundation together with other donors pledged millions for its establishment. It associates diverse members, such as the World Bank, donor country governments, WHO, UNICEF, vaccine manufactures, research agencies, civil society organizations, private sector partners, and implementing country governments. Japan jointed Gavi only in 2011, pledging at the June conference that year, 9.3 million USD in direct contributions for 2011, and maintained a similar annual level until 2014. Aftermath the 2014 Ebola outbreak, Japan doubled its contribution to assist the recovery of health systems. In May 2016, at the G7 leaders' Summit under its presidency, Japan announced a multiyear pledge to Gavi, and in 2019, hosted the launch of Gavi's third replenishment as part of TICAD 7 (Tokyo International Conference on African Development), another Japan's initiative, that occurred in Yokohama (MOFA, 2019).[3]

During the October 2020 Ministerial Meeting of the Group of Friends of UHC, Foreign Minister Motegi reaffirmed Japan's commitment to Gavi and the COVAX AMC initiative. Interestingly, one of the reasons for promoting UHC, as stressed by MOFA in the document prepared for that meeting was that "Japan has been successful in keeping the mortality rate from COVID-19 low because of its strong health system, including its national health insurance scheme" thus putting its health system as a certain model (MOFA, 2020c). Under the scheme, Japan pledged not only to ensure the supply of vaccines through Gavi (USD 300 million, 2021–2025), but also expanding the coverage of diagnostics and therapeutics through the **Global Fund** (USD 840 million for the 2020–2022), another initiative that originated in the G8 Summit in Okinawa in 2000, and furthermore, the capacity building support for the immigration control through JICA, including masks, gloves, thermometers and antiseptics for five countries in Central Asia (MOFA, 2020c).[4] The initiative includes also actions aimed at strengthening resilient and comprehensive health systems in preparation for future health crises, which include reinforcing core medical facilities and networks, regional health systems, improving disease surveillance, and developing human resources and legal frameworks.

Finally, in October 2020, at the Annual meetings of IMF and World Bank Groups, Japan announced a new commitment of 10 million USD to IMF's **COVID-19 Crisis Capacity Development Initiative** to support capacity development activities in low-income countries, with a focus on concrete technical advice on debt management, and a further 10 million USD for International Finance Corporation (IFC) to support Word Bank Group's efforts to ensure equitable and affordable access by all people to health and medical products including vaccines, medicines, and diagnostics (Aso, 2020). Clearly, Japan has been very active in global initiatives.

Domestic vaccination

In the context of the above global efforts, especially regarding immunization, it is interesting to note that domestically Japan was behind the most advanced countries in introducing the vaccines. Moreover, regionally, in comparison to China or India vaccine diplomacy, Japan has been practically invisible. Domestically, the public discussion, concrete laws, programs, and plans for immunization were publicized and introduced only at the end of 2020. There were several reasons behind this apparent delay in the introduction of vaccines in Japan, such as certain "vaccine allergy" exhibits by administrative organs after compensation lawsuits since the 1990s, and following the lack of active engagement of governmental institutions in popularizing immunization, strict procedures for new drug adoption, lack of domestic large pharmaceutical companies, and skeptical public opinion.

First, the Japanese government used to take an active role in developing vaccines such as the combined MMR (measles, mumps, and rubella) vaccine introduced in April 1989, but that changed after a series of lawsuits in the 1990s seeking damages for side effects of the vaccines, which the government lost. After a public outcry fueled by worries over the flu vaccine, the government dropped the requirement for children to be vaccinated against measles or rubella in April 1993 (*The Japan Times*, 14 March 2003, p. 2). In 1999, the government reconsidered using MMR but decided it was safer to keep the ban and continue using individual vaccines for each disease (measles, mumps, and rubella). Since the beginning of the 1990s, there were 3,969 medical compensation claims relating to vaccines, of which a quarter involved side effects of the combined MMR vaccine (Vaccine Confidence Project, 2019). The media thus kept reporting on compensation lawsuits, because many of them continued for years. For instance, in March 2003, the court in Osaka found the government and the Research Foundation of Microbial Diseases of Osaka University responsible for the side effects caused by the MMR vaccine in two cases, ordering to pay a total of 155 million JPY to the families (*The Japan Times*, 14 March 2003, p. 2). In 2010, another series of problems arose concerning HPV vaccination included in the National Immunization Program, which was later terminated in 2013. As a result of the legal defeats, the government did not actively foster the development of new vaccines, neither did it engage in the popularization of immunization. On the other hand, mass media focusing on side effects overemphasized the risks and belittling thereby the benefits of vaccination, contributed to the dissemination of a skeptical outlook on vaccination (Tsukimori, 2021a). Already in the 2014 *Basic Policy on Vaccination*, MHWL emphasized the "vaccine gap" between Japan and other developed countries, pointing to the necessity of raising the rate of immunization, informing and educating the public, as well as fostering the development of domestic vaccines (Kōsei Rōdōshō, 2014: 7–9).

Second, Japanese pharmaceutical companies are comparatively smaller in size due to a lack of consolidation in the sector. Only two (Takeda Pharmaceutical and Astellas Pharma) are among the biggest internationally in terms of revenues, although none of them belongs to the largest five companies that dominate 80% of the global vaccine markets (WHO, 2021b). As a consequence, Japan lags behind in research and development capabilities and international competitiveness (Tsukimori, 2020b). Third, Japan is one of the very few countries that require additional clinical trials within the country to ensure the safety of new drugs. The problem with the COVID-19 vaccine was that with a very low rate of infections, Japan had difficulty in conducting a successful late-stage trial and replicating the high efficacy of the vaccines confirmed overseas. The problem seemed real because of the previous experiences. For instance, after the approval of the Arava rheumatoid arthritis drug in 2003 without conducting a late-stage trial in Japan, 25 patients died out of approximately 5,000 that were administered the drug, and the following investigation revealed that the dosage for the Japanese should have been lower (Tsukimori, 2020a). Nevertheless, in the case of COVID-19, under pressure from Prime Minister Suga, MHWL approved the drug without the last-stage trial within less than two months (Tsukimori, 2021b).

Fourth, the scare of MMR and other vaccines left its mark on the vaccination rate in Japan, as well as the attitudes and perception of risk. Japan has consistently ranked lowest in confidence in vaccines in the world for years. In 2016, a study on vaccine confidence of 67 countries published in *EBioMedicine*, found that 31% of Japanese were skeptical of vaccine safety, ranking third highest following France (45.2%) and Bosnia and Herzegovina (38.3%), while the global average was 13% (Larson et al., 2016: 297). In the most recent polls, the situation has been slightly improving most probably due to the governmental campaigns. The survey conducted by Ipsos in partnership with the World Economic Forum at the end of January 2021 showed that 64% of Japanese respondents were willing to get a vaccine if available, but again Japan was at the lower end, with only France (57%) and Russia (42%) ranking below (Ipsos, 2021: 2). For Japan, that was the 8% increase of "strongly agreeing" (19%) in comparison to the results in December 2020 (Ipsos, 2021: 2). Furthermore, not surprisingly, the percentage of those most concerned with vaccine risk to health (side effects and speed to market) in the same study was the highest in Japan, with 66% worrying about side effects in comparison to European countries, US, Canada or Australia ranging between 31 %(Australia) and 39% (Spain) (Ipsos, 2021: 4). At the same time, it is worth noting that the rate of those against vaccination as such (so-called anti-vaxxers) was among the Japanese very low, 3%, and those concerned that the vaccine was moving through the clinical trials too fast, 14%, much lower than in other countries reflecting the trust in the Japanese approval – long but thorough – procedures (Ipsos, 2021: 4). To tackle the problem of public skepticism, in January 2021, Prime Minister Suga appointed Kōno Tarō, administrative reform minister, who is highly popular among the general public and viewed by many as the next prime minister, to coordinate preparations for delivering the vaccine. Kōno was appointed after the Lower House in November and the Upper House in December 2020 approved a bill to provide free vaccinations against the novel coronavirus to all residents of Japan and placing any liability damages for the pharmaceutical companies on the government. The law includes also a provision obliging citizens to make efforts for getting vaccinated, although it will not go into effect unless the effectiveness and safety of vaccines are fully confirmed. The COVID-19 vaccine was rolled out in Japan in late February 2021, and Kōno was actively engaged in various campaigns aiming at convincing and mobilizing the general public for vaccination.

Conclusion

Japan's response to the COVID-19 pandemic seems at many different levels comparatively successful at the beginning of 2021, both in terms of containment of the pandemic as well as pursuing cooperative relations with other state and non-state actors. There are several factors contributing to that success. Domestically, as mentioned above, Japan had established systemic arrangements long before the pandemic to tackle the public health issues, such as, easy access to medical care under the national health insurance system, and generally high quality of medical care, which help to tackle any health crises. That, together with the Japanese public's high standard of hygiene and other cultural traits, has made Japan better prepared for the occurrence of infectious disease outbreaks. Other factors related to specific measures against COVID-19 include early detection of transmission waves and prompt introduction of countermeasures, Japan's government's comprehensive involvement in tackling the infection outbreak, as well as the government's reliance on experts' opinions when making crucial decisions. All these measures have clearly helped to contain the spread of the coronavirus and mitigate its impact. Japan government's response was not unusual, however, in the sense that it reflected its highly centralized political system, previous practices, and political culture, in which the government is expected to take initiative, responsibility, and at least partial control. Regarding securing supplies necessary for health and medical products, the government included them into the strategic commodities launching a variety of programs to increase domestic production, foster reshoring, and nearshoring, such as Subsidy Project for Supporting Businesses in Introducing Facilities for Producing Face Masks, Subsidy Project for Supporting Businesses in Introducing Facilities for Producing Protective Clothing, Subsidy Project for Supporting Businesses in Introducing Facilities for Producing Ventilators and Other Medical Equipment, and finally Program for Promoting Investment in Japan to Strengthen Supply Chains. It is important to note that the division of commodities into strategic and nonstrategic precedes the pandemic. The rise of China and the most recent US-China trade war made Japan's government sensitive to the vulnerability of supply chains and began the process of designating some products (e.g., semiconductors, telecommunications) as critical and strategic some years ago.

Second, on the regional level, Japan's response was probably the most complex, essentially cooperative but also clearly divided into strategic and nonstrategic cooperation. For the strategic commodities, Japan decided to diversify or/and shift production sites to countries that are Japan's allies or partners in important initiatives, such as FOIP and QUAD, to secure critical supply chains. One of the projects that JETRO launched during the pandemic was the Program for Strengthening Overseas Supply Chains, assisting the shift of Japanese companies to ASEAN, which again fits into the earlier China Plus One supply chain management strategy. Another example of this trend is the Resilient Supply Chain Initiative (RSCI) signed between Japan, Australia, and India. At the same time, it worth remembering that Japan's decisions to secure certain products do not imply a decoupling of Japan's economy from China in a broader strategic sense. China is too close to Japan and too big a market to be ignored. Even during the pandemic Japan continued its activities aimed at enhancing regional cooperation, participating in such events as the Special ASEAN Plus Three Summit on Coronavirus Disease 2019 (COVID-19), the Special ASEAN Plus Three Economic Ministers' Virtual Conference Meeting on COVID-19 Response, and finally also signing Regional Comprehensive Economic Partnership (RCEP) in November 2020 together with China, Australia, and other countries.

Third, on the global level, Japan became deeply involved in several important COVID-19 initiatives of WHO, IMF, World Bank, and other institutions, including IMF's Catastrophe Containment and Relief Trust (CCRT), IMF's Poverty Reduction and Growth Trust (PRGT), IMF's COVID-19 Crisis Capacity Development Initiative, International Finance Corporation (IFC) of World Bank Group, Global Vaccine Summit, Gavi and COVAX AMC. Japan initiated some time ago a program of Universal Health Coverage (UHC), which was fostered during the pandemic and embedded into other COVID-19-related undertakings. Therefore, on the global level, Japan's activities can be categorized as highly cooperative, and proactive, reflecting its policy of multilateralism and global cooperation.

Finally, it is worth emphasizing that although the impact of COVID-19 on Japan's public health and economy has been substantial and undeniable, it has not fundamentally changed health, security, or economic policies, but rather accelerated earlier trends caused by the growing power of China and the hegemonic rivalry with the United States. Japan, as a very close and loyal ally of the USA, has therefore chosen to deepen strategic cooperation aimed at securing the supply chains of critical goods under the FOIP, QUAD, and other frameworks with its allies and like-minded partners. However, it should be kept in mind that in the process of restructuring the cross-border production networks, reshoring and nearshoring some of them from China to ASEAN and other places, other economic factors, such as labor and transport costs, also play an important role. Therefore, it is more accurate to perceive it as a convergence of geopolitical and market-driven economic factors in shaping the behavior of Japanese companies rather than only as the result of the pandemic or rising of the US-China rivalry. Furthermore, due to the geographical proximity, size, and power of China's market, Japan has promoted a variety of regional cooperation frameworks engaging its powerful neighbor, and little change in this respect can be expected. The main difference in the post-COVID-19 world might be a clear distinction between strategic and nonstrategic cooperation. Severe competition, alienation, containment, decoupling, or de-linking from the world's second-largest economy and the main trading partner is not an option for Japan while developing strategic and non-nonstrategic cooperative relations certainly is.

References

ASEAN (2020), *Ha Noi Declaration on The Fifteenth Anniversary of The East Asia Summit*, 14 November 2020, https://asean.org/storage/2020/11/29-Ha-Noi-Declaration-on-the-15th-Anniversary-of-the-EAS-FINAL.pdf, (Accessed: 17.2.2021).

Aso T. (2020), *Statement by the Hon. TARO ASO, Governor of the Bank for Japan*, 15 October 2020, https://www.worldbank.org/content/dam/meetings/external/annualmeeting-1/WBGS202010-Japan-E-final.pdf, (Accessed: 17.2.2021).

Cabinet Secretariat (2020), *28th Meeting of the Novel Coronavirus Response Headquarters*, 11 April 2020, https://japan.kantei.go.jp/98_abe/actions/202004/_00013.html, (Accessed: 16.2.2021).

David D. (2020), 'Japan's experience in reducing its supply chain insecurity', *Asia Power Watch*, 12 October 2020, https://asiapowerwatch.com/japans-experience-in-reducing-its-supply-chain-insecurity/, (Accessed: 17.2.2020).

Gavi (2020a), COVAX AMC, https://www.gavi.org/gavi-covax-amc, (Accessed: 17.2.2021).

Gavi (2020b), *Donor Profiles: Japan*, 26 March 2020, https://www.gavi.org/investing-gavi/funding/donor-profiles/japan, (Accessed: 17.2.2021).

Hale T., Webster S., Petherick A., Phillips T., Kira B. (2020), *Oxford COVID-19 Government Response Tracker. COVID-19: Government Stringency Index*, Blavatnik School of Government, https://www.bsg.ox.ac.uk/research/research-projects/coronavirus-government-response-tracker, (Accessed: 15.2. 2021).

Hosoya Y. (2019), *FOIP 2.0: The Evolution of Japan's Free and Open Indo-Pacific Strategy,*"Asia-Pacific Review", 26 (1), pp. 18–28.

IMF (2020), *Japan Boosts its Contributions to IMF's Catastrophe Relief Fund and Poverty Reduction and Growth Trust*, April 30, 2020, https://www.imf.org/en/News/Articles/2020/04/30/pr20197-japan-boosts-contributions-imf-catastrophe-relief-fund-poverty-reduction-growth-trust, (Accessed: 10.2.2021).

Ipsos (2021), *Global Attitudes on a COVID-19 Vaccine*, https://www.ipsos.com/sites/default/files/Global-attitudes-on-a-COVID-19-Vaccine-January-2021-report%20.pdf, (Accessed: 15.2.2021).

JETRO (Japan External Trade Organization) (2020), *Program for Strengthening Overseas Supply Chains*, https://www.jetro.go.jp/ext_images/services/supply-chain/kekka1_en.pdf, (Accessed: 17.2.2021).

Johnson C. A. (1985), *MITI and the Japanese miracle: The growth of industrial policy, 1925–1975*, Stanford: Stanford University Press.

Kantei (2020a), *25th Meeting of the Novel Coronavirus Response Headquarters*, 1 April 2020, https://japan.kantei.go.jp/98_abe/actions/202004/_00001.html, (Accessed: 17.2.2021).

Kantei (2020b), *Emergency Economic Measures for Response to COVID-19 to protect the lives and lifestyles of the public and move toward economic recovery*, 20 April 2020, http://japan.kantei.go.jp/ongoingtopics/_00019.html, (Accessed: 16.2.2021).

Kantei (2020c), *Shingata Koronauirusu Kansenshō Taisaku Senmonka Kaigi (dai 11-kai), Shingata koronauirusu Kansenshō Taisaku no Jōkyō Bunseki Teigen* [Novel Coronavirus Expert Meeting (11th meeting) Analysis and recommendations for countermeasures for new coronavirus infections], 22 April 2020, https://www.kantei.go.jp/jp/singi/novel_coronavirus/senmonkakaigi/sidai_r020422.pdf, (Accessed: 16.1.2021).

Keisatsuchō [National Police Agency] (2021), *Reiwa 2-nen no tsugibetsu jisatsushasū ni tsuite* [Number of suicides by month in 2020], 31 January 2021, https://www.npa.go.jp/safetylife/seianki/jisatsu/R02/zantei0212.pdf, (Accessed: 18.2.2021).

Kezai Sangyōshō [Ministry of Economy, Trade and Industry] (2020a), *Reiwa 2-nen-do 'Bōgofuku Seisan Setsubi Dōnyū Shien Jigyō' no Saitaku Kekka ni Tsuite* [Selection result of 'Protective clothing production equipment introduction support project' 2020], 18 May 2020, https://www.meti.go.jp/information/publicoffer/saitaku/2020/s200518001.html, (Accessed: 17.2.2021).

Kezai Sangyōshō [Ministry of Economy, Trade and Industry] (2020b), *Reiwa 2-nen-do 'Jinkō Kokyūki tō Seisan Setsubi Dōnyū Shien Hojo Jigyō' no Saitaku Kekka ni Tsuite* [Selection results of 'Reiwa production equipment introduction support assistance project' 2020], 19 May 2020, https://www.meti.go.jp/information/publicoffer/saitaku/2020/s200519001.html, (Accessed: 17.2.2021).

Kōsei Rōdōshō [Ministry of Health, Welfare and Labour] (2014), *Yobō sesshu ni kansuru kihon-tekina keikaku* [Basic plan for vaccination], 28 March 2014, https://www.mhlw.go.jp/bunya/kenkou/kekkaku-kansenshou20/dl/yobou140529–1.pdf, (Accessed: 17.2.2021).

Kōsei Rōdōshō [Ministry of Health, Welfare and Labour] (2020–2021), *Shingata Koronauirusu Kansenbyō Taisaku Adobaizarībōdo no shiryō tō* [Documents of the Novel Coronavirus Advisory Board], https://www.mhlw.go.jp/stf/seisaku-nitsuite/bunya/0000121431_00093.html, (Accessed: 15.2.2021).

Kōsei Rōdōshō [Ministry of Health, Welfare and Labour] (2020a), *Jinko dōtai tōkei sokuhō (gaisū) (Heisei 28 nen – Reiwa 2 nen)* [Monthly vital statistics report (Approximate number) (2016–2020)], https://www.mhlw.go.jp/content/10700000/sanko2.pdf, (Accessed: 18.2.2021).

Kōsei Rōdōshō [Ministry of Health, Welfare and Labour] (2020b), *Shingata Koronauirusu Kansenbyō Taisaku Adobaizarībōdo (dai 3 kai) giji gaiyō* [Novel Coronavirus Advisory Board (Third meeting) minutes summary], https://www.mhlw.go.jp/content/10900000/000681424.pdf, (Accessed: 6.2.2021).

Kōsei Rōdōshō [Ministry of Health, Welfare and Labour] (2020c), *Yokohama minato de ken'eki o okonatta kurūzusen ni kanren shita kanja no shibō ni tsuite* [death of a patient related to a cruise ship quarantined at Yokohama Port], https://www.mhlw.go.jp/stf/newpage_10870.html, (Accessed: 6.2.2021).

Larson H. J., de Figueiredo A, Xiahong Z, et al. (2016), *The State of Vaccine Confidence 2016: Global Insights Through a 67-Country Survey*,"EBioMedicine", 12: 295–301.

METI (2008), *The White Paper on International Economy and Trade 2008*, https://www.meti.go.jp/english/report/data/gWT2008fe.html, (Accessed: 18.2.2021).

METI (2020a), *ASEAN Plus Three Economic Ministers' Joint Statement on Mitigating the Economic Impact of the COVID-19 Pandemic Issued*, 4 June 2020, https://www.meti.go.jp/english/press/2020/0604_002.html, (Accessed: 17.2.2021).

METI (2020b), *Australia-India-Japan Economic Ministers' Joint Statement on Supply Chain Resilience*, 1 September 2020, https://www.meti.go.jp/press/2020/09/20200901008/20200901008–1.pdf, (Accessed: 17.2.2021).

METI (2020c), *Certificates of Gratitude Granted to Companies and Associations that Contributed to Increase in Production of Medical Supplies*, 21 Dec. 2020, https://www.meti.go.jp/english/press/2020/1221_002.html, (Accessed: 17.2.2021).

METI (2020d), *Companies to be Subsidized under the FY2019 Subsidy Project for Supporting Businesses in Introducing Facilities for Producing Face Masks Nominated*, 19 May 2020, https://www.meti.go.jp/english/press/2020/0313_002.html, (Accessed: 17.2.2021).

METI (2020e), *Current Status of Production and Supply of Face Masks, Antiseptics and Toilet Paper*, 19 May 2020, https://www.meti.go.jp/english/covid-19/mask.html, (Accessed: 17.2.2021).

METI (2020f), *Successful Applicants Selected for the Program for Promoting Investment in Japan to Strengthen Supply Chains*, 20 November 2020, https://www.meti.go.jp/english/press/2020/1120_001.html, (Accessed: 17.2.2021).

MHWL (2021a) *Novel Coronavirus (COVID-19), Overview*, https://www.mhlw.go.jp/stf/seisakunitsuite/bunya/0000164708_00079.html, (Accessed: 15.2.2021).

MHWL (2021b), *Current situation in Japan*, 17 February 2021, https://www.mhlw.go.jp/stf/covid-19/kokunainohasseijoukyou_00006.html#1–1, (Accessed: 15.2.2021).

Midford, P. (2020), *Overcoming Isolationism: Japan's Leadership in East Asian Security Multilateralism*, Stanford University Press.

MOF (Ministry of Finance) (2021), *Highlights of the FY2021 Draft Budget*, January 2021, https://www.mof.go.jp/english/budget/budget/fy2021/01.pdf, (Accessed: 18.2.2021).

MOFA (Ministry of Foreign Affairs) (2019), *The Seventh Tokyo International Conference on African Development (TICAD7)*, 26 November 2019, https://www.mofa.go.jp/afr/af2/page25e_000274.html, (Accessed: 17.2.2021).

MOFA (Ministry of Foreign Affairs) (2020a), *Address by Prime Minister Suga at the Seventy-Fifth Session of the United Nations General Assembly*, 16 September 2020, https://www.mofa.go.jp/fp/unp_a/page4e_001095.html, (Accessed: 17.2.2021).

MOFA (Ministry of Foreign Affairs) (2020b), *Japan-Australia Leaders' Meeting Joint Statement*, 17 November 2020, https://www.mofa.go.jp/files/100116180.pdf, (Accessed: 17.2.2021).

MOFA (Ministry of Foreign Affairs) (2020c), *Japanese cooperation to "Leave No One's Health Behind" – towards achieving Universal Health Coverage (UHC)*, October 2020, https://www.mofa.go.jp/files/100101479.pdf, (Accessed: 17.2.2021).

MOFA (Ministry of Foreign Affairs) (2020d), *Minister MOTEGI Toshimitsu co-hosted Ministerial Meeting of Group of Friends of Universal Health Coverage (UHC)*, 8 October 2020, https://www.mofa.go.jp/press/release/press4e_002929.html, (Accessed: 17.2.2021).

MOFA (Ministry of Foreign Affairs) (2020e), *Special ASEAN Plus Three (Japan-China-ROK) Summit on Coronavirus Disease 2019 (COVID-19)*, 14 April 2020.

Nagy S. R. (2020a), *Accommodation versus Alliance: Japan's Prospective Grand Strategy in the Sino-US Competition*, "The Asan Forum", 27 August, http://www.theasanforum.org/accommodation-versus-alliance-japans-prospective-grand-strategy-in-the-sino-us-competition/, (Accessed: 18.2.2021).

Nagy S. R. (2020b), *Maritime Cooperation between Middle Powers in the Indo-Pacific: Aligning Interests with Capability and Capacity*, "Issues and Insights" 20, No. 1 (working paper, Pacific-Forum, March): 1–6.

Nagy S. R. (2021), Author's online interview, 19 February 2021.

Nakafuji R. (2019), *Quarter of Japanese companies ready to reduce China footprint*, "Nikkei Asia", 4 October 2020, https://asia.nikkei.com/Economy/Trade-war/

Quarter-of-Japanese-companies-ready-to-reduce-China-footprint, (Accessed: 17.2.2021).

NHK (2020a), *Naikaku Shijiritsu* [Cabinet support rate], 14 April 2020, https://www.nhk.or.jp/senkyo/shijiritsu/archive/2020_04.html, (Accessed: 16.2.2021).

NHK (2020b), *Naikaku Shijiritsu* [Cabinet support rate], 14 July 2020, https://www.nhk.or.jp/senkyo/shijiritsu/archive/2020_07.html, (Accessed: 16.2.2021).

NHK (2020c), *Naikaku Shijiritsu* [Cabinet support rate], 15 December 2020, https://www.nhk.or.jp/senkyo/shijiritsu/archive/2020_12.html, (Accessed: 16.2.2021).

NHK (2021), *Naikaku Shijiritsu* [Cabinet support rate], Feb. 8, 2021, https://www.nhk.or.jp/senkyo/shijiritsu/, (Accessed: 17.2.2021).

NNA Business News (3 June 2019), *Teikoku Databank survey: Some Japanese firms leaving China on uncertain growth outlook,* https://english.nna.jp/articles/886, (Accessed: 17.2.2021).

Nōrin Suisanshō [Ministry of Agriculture, Forestry and Fisheries] (2019), *Sekai no shokuryō jikyūritsu* [World food self-sufficiency rate], as of 2019, https://www.maff.go.jp/j/zyukyu/zikyu_ritu/013.html, (Accessed: 18.2.2021).

Omi S., Oshitani H. (2020), *Japan's COVID-19 Response*, 1 June 2020, https://corona.go.jp/en/news/pdf/COVID19Response_20200602.pdf, (Accessed: 22.1.2021).

Oshitani H. (2020), *Cluster-Based Approach to Coronavirus Disease 2019 (COVID-19) Response in Japan, from February to April 2020*, "Laboratory and Epidemiology Communications", 73: 491–493.

Our World in Data (2021), *Total confirmed COVID-19 deaths and cases per million people,* https://ourworldindata.org/grapher/total-covid-cases-deaths-per-million?yScale=log&time=2019–12–31..latest, (Accessed: 15.2.2021).

Palit A. (2020), *The Resilient Supply Chain Initiative: Reshaping Economics Through Geopolitics,* "The Diplomat", 10 September 2020, https://thediplomat.com/2020/09/the-resilient-supply-chain-initiative-reshaping-economics-through-geopolitics/, (Accessed: 17.2.2021).

Soeya Y. (2020), *Middle-Power Cooperation in the Indo-Pacific Era*, "Issues & Studies", 56 (2), https://www.worldscientific.com/doi/abs/10.1142/S1013251120400093, (Accessed: 8.2.2021).

Takeo Y. and M. Jamrisko (2020), *Japan Push to Cut China Reliance May Be Boost for Southeast Asia*, "Bloomberg", 10 August 2020, https://www.bloombergquint.com/business/japan-push-to-cut-china-reliance-may-be-boost-for-southeast-asia, (Accessed: 17.2.2021).

The Japan Times (17 Dec. 2020), *Japan's review of Avigan as COVID-19 treatment draws blank*, "The Japan Times", https://www.japantimes.co.jp/news/2020/12/17/national/science-health/japan-avigan-review/, (Accessed: 17.2.2021).

Tsukimori O. (2020a), *Not so fast, Japan experts say, as COVID-19 vaccines raise hopes*, "The Japan Times", 25 November 2020, https://www.japantimes.co.jp/

news/2020/11/25/national/science-health/japan-experts-coronavirus-vaccines-safety/, (Accessed: 17.2.2021).

Tsukimori O. (2020b), *Why Japan is largely a spectator in the coronavirus vaccine race,* "The Japan Times", 11 December 2020, https://www.japantimes.co.jp/news/2020/12/11/business/japan-slow-corona-vaccine/, (Accessed: 17.2.2021).

Tsukimori O. (2021a), *Japan scrambles to roll out vaccine, but how many people will get the shot?,* "The Japan Times", 18 January 2021, https://www.japantimes.co.jp/news/2021/01/18/national/science-health/coronavirus-vaccine-skeptics/, (Accessed: 17.2.2021).

Tsukimori O. (2021b), *Japan prepares to dispense Pfizer vaccine from Wednesday after formal approval,* "The Japan Times", February 2021, https://www.japantimes.co.jp/news/2021/02/15/national/science-health/pfizer-vaccine-approval-japan/, (Accessed: 17.2.2021).

Vaccine Confidence Project (2019), *Japan: Why Japan banned MMR vaccine,* 11 May 2019, https://www.vaccineconfidence.org/latest-news/japan-why-japan-banned-mmr-vaccine, (Accessed: 17.2.2021).

WHO (2020a), *Interim Guidancel,* 10 January 2020, https://apps.who.int/iris/bitstream/handle/10665/332447/WHO-2019-nCoV-IPC-2020.1-eng.pdf, (Accessed: 3.2.2021).

WHO (2020b), *Vaccine market, Global Vaccine Supply,* https://www.who.int/immunization/programmes_systems/procurement/market/global_supply/en/, (Accessed: 17.2.2021).

WHO (2021), *Timeline: WHO's COVID-19 response,* https://www.who.int/emergencies/diseases/novel-coronavirus-2019/interactive-timeline#!, (Accessed: 17.2.2021).

Artur Pohl
Adam Mickiewicz University, Poznan
ORCID: 0000-0002-2975-0425

COVID-19 RESPONSE IN SOUTH AMERICA. THE CASE OF BRAZIL AND CHILE[1]

Globalization and the associated technological development, making it possible to travel long distances faster, have eliminated the natural geographic limitations of the spread of infectious diseases. The intensification of trade exchange and strengthening of international cooperation of companies from different regions, as well as ordinary tourist trips to distant corners of the world, mean that within a few hours pathogens found in one part of the world can spread to many others. It is no different with the SARS-CoV-2 coronavirus (Severe Acute Respiratory Syndrome Coronavirus 2), causing the COVID-19 disease, which from China, among others across Europe, reached distant South America[2].

The first case of COVID-19 was confirmed in Brazil on February 26 in a patient who a few days earlier had returned from a trip to Lombardy in northern Italy (Rodriguez-Morales, Gallego, Escalera-Antezana, et al., 2020; De Sousa, Savarese, 2020). Since then, the spread of the epidemic in South America has gathered pace, and further cases of infection with the virus were also reported in Ecuador and Chile, and then in the rest of the region. By the end of 2020, the number of detected SARS-CoV-2 infections in all countries of the region exceeded 13 million, and 360,000 fatalities (*14-day COVID-19, 2021; Covid-19 Coronavirus Pandemic, 2021*). At the same time, however,

---

[1] The research was financed from the project „Research on COVID-19" from the funds of the Adam Mickiewicz University, Poznan

[2] South America will be understood as the area of 14 countries: Argentina, Bolivia, Brazil, Chile, Colombia, Ecuador, Falkland Islands, Guyana, French Guiana, Paraguay, Peru, Suriname, Uruguay, and Venezuela.

it should be emphasized that the possibility of comparing statistical data – published by the governments of individual countries and then used by institutions and organizations compiling the lists – is limited. It is related to, inter alia, the methodology of data collection, but also to differences, e.g. in the number of tests performed. It is also worth noting that the development of the epidemic in individual countries of the region varied significantly, as they faced different challenges related to social, economic, and political problems, as well as international and health policy. Although the region of South America may appear to be relatively homogeneous, it is only an impression. As in other parts of the world, the countries of this region differ in terms of the structure of society, the degree of urbanization and population density, the level of economic development, climate, the level of financing of the health service or the discipline of the population, the political system, and many other factors. The analysis of the above-mentioned determinants and health policies carried out in the face of the Covid-19 pandemic in 2020 by all South American countries, as well as their impact on international relations, significantly exceeds the scope of this article, therefore the author will focus on the study of only two states: Brazil and Chile. This choice is dictated primarily by the significant difference between the actions taken by the political leaders of the first country and the generally accepted pattern of conduct. In the case of the latter, an important premise is the relatively high representativeness of data compared to other countries in the region, associated with a large number of tests per million inhabitants. This article will focus both on the presentation of the reactions of the above-mentioned states to the threat and on international cooperation within the framework of existing regional organizations.

Institutional regional cooperation in the field of health policy

The idea of integrating South America dates back to the times of decolonization and independence gained by the countries of the region, which started a discussion on the political future of the continent. Since then, many initiatives have been created to strengthen cooperation and ties in this area, but also to raise its role in the international arena. Due to numerous problems and threats to the health of the region's societies, the need for transnational cooperation has also covered the sphere of health policy, therefore it is considered as an important element of many integration mechanisms, including intergovernmental organizations. As early as 1873, due to increased immigration to the coastal cities of the Empire of Brazil and the Republics of Uruguay and Argentina, these countries decided to standardize the hitherto differential quarantine measures in order to protect the population, but also to unify the regulations on trade, primarily in the food sector, protecting themselves against "exotic epidemics"[3] which came with migrants. The need to institutionalize cooperation in the field of health between the countries of the Western hemisphere was reflected in the Pan American Health Organization (PAHO) established in 1902[4], which is now a component of both the World Health Organization (WHO) and the inter-American system[5] (Herraro & Tussie, 2015: 263–264). Latin American states have also assigned competencies in the field of health to other international organizations and mechanisms they have established, including the Common Market of the South (Mercado Común del Sur – MERCOSUR), the Andean Health Organization, and the Union of South American Nations (Unión de Naciones Suramericanas – UNASUR) and the Forum for the Progress and Integration of South America (Foro para el Progreso e Integración de América del Sur – PROSUR). At the same time, South American countries are members of global organizations which, in their missions and goals, also have the sphere of health protection: WHO and the International Monetary Fund (IMF).

The development of the pandemic caused by the SARS-CoV-2 virus meant that the above-mentioned international cooperation forums have become an even more important element of active health policy in the region. The mechanisms they activate are aimed at supporting and coordinating actions taken by the governing bodies of individual member states, including their co-financing, as well as facilitating the exchange of information related to the spread of the virus.

---

[3] I. a. Cholera and yellow fever.

[4] At the time, it functioned as the International Sanitary Bureau, renamed the Pan-American Sanitary Bureau at the Fifth International Conference of American States in Santiago de Chile in 1923 (Minor, 1941: 45). It was included in the structure of the *Constitution of the Pan American Sanitary Organization*, 1947, established in 1947, which had been renamed to the Pan-American Health Organization in 1958 during the 15th Pan-American Sanitary Conference (De Lima, Bruera, 2000).

[5] As the WHO Regional Office for the Americas, a specialized health agency within the Organization of American States – as defined in Chapter XVIII of the Charter of the Organization of American States (De Lima, Bruera, 2000; *Specialized*, 2021),

As a response to the resulting threat, PAHO decided to launch multi-vector activities aimed at preventing the spread of SARS-CoV-2 in the Americas. The organization has developed a number of technical guidelines and documents supporting the development of strategies and policies in the era of a pandemic, e.g. indicating ways of maintaining safety in pandemic conditions (even as a result of natural disasters), water treatment and hygiene, methods of detecting and reporting infections, monitoring of health care system load or travel-related procedures (see more: *Technical Documents*, 2021). The organization also launched the COVID-19 information system for the Americas region - Geo-Hub (https://paho-covid19-response-who. hub.arcgis.com), which publishes the latest data on the development of the epidemic in the Western Hemisphere, including on daily illnesses, trends, and the reproduction rate of the virus, as well as reports on the actions taken by countries (*Coronavirus Disease*, 2021), and also works towards integrating COVID-19 information in the surveillance system for severe acute respiratory diseases / flu-like diseases - SARI / ILI systems (*COVID-19 - PAHO / WHO*, 2020). The cooperation of American countries within PAHO also included activities related to training for personnel in the field of testing, case tracking, and patient care. The established PAHO Response Fund for COVID-19, under which USD 263 million was collected from various donors in 2020[6], allowed to finance 224 such training, and also send over 21.4 million PCR tests to Member States (Epstein, Nusser, 2021) as well as personal protective equipment: 3 million pairs of gloves, 36 million respiratory and surgical masks, 365 thousand pairs of goggles and nearly 2 million gowns (*The PAHO COVID-19*, 2021; *COVID-19 - PAHO / WHO*, 2020). The organization also works to promote, educate and support the vaccination process against the virus, including logistics and providing access to vaccines.

Cooperation in the fight against COVID-19 between the countries of South America is also carried out under the aegis of organizations related only to this region. Although Mercosur was established[7] with the aim of economic integration – creating a common market, health issues were also taken into account in the thematic scope of the activities undertaken. The organization – through meetings of health ministers – is a political forum where the health policies of the Member States and associated countries are

---

[6] Part of the funds was financed by technical support

[7] Pursuant to the Treaty of Asunción, concluded on March 26, 1991, the contracting parties agreed to establish a common market by December 31, 1994.

harmonized, but also a technical forum – meetings of working groups – where national standards and regulations in medical sector related to the free movement of goods, people and services are harmonized (e.g. blood, blood derivatives, drugs, pharmaceuticals, medical products, health services, border controls, technological processes) (Aneiros Fernandez et. al., 2013: 26). The outbreak of the COVID-19 pandemic posed serious challenges for MERCOSUR related to decisions taken by the Member States to close borders, limit the flow of people, services, and products – severe for cross-border cities and communities operating in border zones, in particular – but also opened new perspectives for accelerating the process integration. First, the organization is a forum for discharging emerging cross-border tensions and disputes resulting from unilateral actions by governments. On March 18, 2020, Member States decided to adopt *the MERCOSUR Presidents' Declaration on regional coordination in combating the coronavirus and mitigating its impact* (*Declaracion*, 2020). Second, the temporary suspension or restriction of the freedom of movement of people, goods, and services agreed under MERCOSUR may visualize or remind South American elites and societies what are the advantages of deepened integration. Thirdly, the organization's response to the consequences of a pandemic, such as an economic slowdown, increased debt, or unemployment, may turn out to be crucial for the economic situation of individual Member States. So far, in response to the development of the pandemic, the MERCOSUR group within the existing Structural Convergence Fund, which includes the project "Research, education, and health-applied biotechnologies", redirected some funds in March 2020 – 520 thousand USD – for activities supporting the infection detection process[8], and established, at the beginning of April, an additional, non-returnable, and interest-free emergency fund of nearly USD 16 million to fight COVID-19,[9] increased in October by additional funds for Argentina (over USD 1 million) and Uruguay (less than $ 2.5 million) (*Salud*, 2021).

Another platform for cooperation in the fight against the COVID-19 pandemic, involving Bolivia, Chile, Ecuador, Colombia, Peru, and Vene-

---

[8] Equipment, reagents, personal protective equipment, virus detection kits.

[9] To strengthen the diagnostic potential, purchase of equipment and personal protective equipment, and tests for the rapid detection of virus infections. The fund is also intended to support the development of a serological diagnostic technique that allows the detection of antibodies in symptomatic and asymptomatic people, which will allow the degree of viral penetration in society to be determined.

zuela, is the Andean Health Organization.[10] It is an institution that in 1998 was included in the Andean Integration System,[11] organized under the auspices of the Andean Community, the aim of which is to promote the sustainable and harmonious development of the Member States on the basis of equality through economic and social integration and cooperation, accelerating their economic growth, creating new workplaces, and to facilitate their participation in the process of regional integration, which is to lead to the gradual establishment of the Latin American common market (*Acuerdo de Integracion*, 1969: Art. 1). For the western states of South American the Andean Health Organization has become a forum for consultation and cooperation of their health policies in the field of combating COVID-19. The organization publish on its website information on the development of the pandemic in the world and in the Andean region, educational materials on behavior in pandemic, which help to protect one's own and others' physical and mental health, as well as adresses of websites containing the most important information related to the virus, compiled by national institutions (*Covid-19. ¿Que es*, 2021). The organization also supports individual member states in developing actions to improve health in a pandemic situation, and above all provides a platform for political and technical meetings during which information on research into the virus and how to combat it is exchanged.

As late as 2018, the Union of South American Nations had significant potential to coordinate activities and undertake cooperation in the field of health by all the independent states of the continent. One of its main tasks was the cultural, social, economic, and political integration of the entire continent (MERCOSUR, Andean Community, Chile, Suriname, and Guyana) through political dialogue, social, educational, energy, infrastructure, financial, and environmental policies (*Tratado Constitutivo*,2008: Art. 2). One of the priorities of UNASUR was health policy, whose coordination and strengthening was appointed by the South American Council of Health, which takes actions in particular in the areas of detecting and responding to health problems, development of universal health systems, social determinants of health, universal access to medicine, and the development of medical staff (more: Herraro, Tussie, 2015: 269). However, the significant potential of UNASUR to tighten cooperation between states, create a com-

---

[10] Earlier, the Agreement of Hippolyte Unanuego.

[11] Pursuant to Decision 445 of the Andean Council of Foreign Ministers (*Decision 445*, 1998).

mon platform for protecting public health, and fight threats to it – resulting from focusing on social problems – paradoxically has also become a cause of the disintegration of the institution. The transfer of power to right-wing and center-right groups in many South American countries made the rulers reluctant to continue the integration initiated by their left-wing and center-left predecessors within the Union of South American States and launched a competitive project – PROSUR (*Mausoleum,* 2019). As part of the Forum for the Progress and Development of South America, Member States have identified health as one of the key integration areas, alongside infrastructure, energy, defense, security and crime-fighting, and disaster crisis management (*Informe*, 2020: 6). The outbreak of the COVID-19 pandemic meant that cooperation in the fight against this threat and its consequences has become one of the main problems for a relatively young institution. This can be considered both an obstacle but also an extraordinary opportunity for the acceleration of integration, coordination of activities, and cooperation by highlighting the advantages of cooperation over unilateral proceedings. From March to December 2020, as part of PROSUR, four meetings at the summit with the participation of heads of state were devoted to COVID-19 issues. They ended with the adoption of three declarations on joint actions aimed at counteracting the threat. They identified five key areas for cooperation, called work tables:

1. Movement of people – informing about the requirements, regulations, and documents necessary for crossing borders between PROSUR countries, standardizing procedures related to migration, as well as coordinating the process of re-opening borders;
2. Epidemiology and data – comparison and exchange of information on the methods and effects of detecting and fighting an epidemic, as well as data on its development, which is to support the decision-making process by the relevant state authorities;
3. Joint purchases – creating a mechanism for joint purchasing of medical products (equipment, drugs, etc.) – primarily with the use of existing PAHO instruments. Submitting a demand as a grouping is to strengthen the competitiveness and purchasing power of PROSUR countries on the international market;
4. Movement of goods – exchange of pandemic-related information on regulations and restrictions on the movement of goods across borders in each PROSUR country to guarantee the freedom of export and import of goods;

5. Access to international loans and funds – supporting member states (whose economies have found themselves in a difficult situation as a result of measures taken to combat COVID-19) in obtaining international funds and loans for support from institutions such as the Inter-American Development Bank, the Development Bank of Latin American (*Informe*, 2020: 22–25).

The potential of PROSUR, as it was the case with UNASUR before, to strengthen international cooperation in the region is significant – also in the field of health policies. It should be noted, however, that a deeper and lasting process of South American integration will not take place as long as the ideological rivalry between the left and the right will lead to a continual start again – building new projects, and not continuing the existing ones.[12]

However, the fight against COVID-19 was undertaken primarily at the level of individual countries. Their unilateral actions constitute the basic form of counteracting the development of a pandemic and its consequences. Moreover, the state authorities are predestined to pursue health policies and have in their hands the appropriate tools to limit the spread of the virus and provide adequate care for patients suffering from SARS-CoV-2. Nevertheless, the nature of the threat that knows no national borders, as well as the effects of the actions taken, have an international dimension, and unilateral decisions and strategies to combat COVID-19 should support and be supported by multilateral ones. It is important because coordinated and standardized procedures, in particular globally and regionally, can more effectively influence the fight against the pandemic and the elimination of its effects. However, not all state authorities decided to react to the threat as was recommended by international institutions. Countries have adopted various strategies in this regard – also in South America. Therefore it seems worthy taking a closer look at the health policies of Brazil and Chile, which differ fundamentally.

Covid-19 and health policy against the epidemic in Brazil

The first case of COVID-19 infection in South America was confirmed in Brazil – the most populous and largest – also in the context of the economy

---

[12] As for UNASUR and PROSUR.

– country in the region,.[13] However, it is another factor that makes it worth taking a closer look at the development of the epidemic situation and the response to it in this country. The federal authorities, headed by President Jaire Bolsonaro, have chosen a strategy of dealing with the threat that is different from that of most countries in the world and the region.

Taking into account the previous experiences and actions taken by the Brazilian authorities to improve the quality of health care and increase its potential to fight HIV or Zika viruses, one could hope that also in the case of COVID-19, the state would rise to the challenge and become a model for other countries (Londoño, Andreoni, Casado, 2020a). It was all the more justified because, in 2018 in Brazil, slightly more than 9.5% of GDP was allocated to health care, which put it in the lead of the region, just behind Argentina (9.62% of GDP), and before Uruguay (9.2 % Of GDP) and Chile (9.14% of GDP). Also, taking into account healthcare expenditure per capita per year, Brazil is among the leaders in South America, but only in fourth place – behind the above-mentioned states[14] (The World Bank, 2021). Although it might seem that relatively high investment in health care should be an undoubted advantage in the fight against SARS-CoV-2, these indicators do not directly translate into the effectiveness of risk elimination, as shown also by examples of richer countries. Nevertheless, the statistics on the disease coming from Brazil are extremely worrying and make the country be viewed as one of the centers of the epidemic's development. By the end of 2020, nearly 7 million 700 thousand cases of COVID-19 infections (the third-highest number in the world) and almost 200,000 deaths as a consequence of the disease (the second-highest number in the world) were recorded in the country[15]. Equally pessimistic and daring to look to the future, the figures were for the daily number of new cases – 55,853 and 56,003 – and deaths – 1,224 and 1,036 – on December 30 and 31, respectively (*Covid-19 Coronavirus Pandemic*, 2021).

When looking for the reasons for such a dynamic development of the epidemic in Brazil, it is impossible not to pay attention to the politics and rhetoric conducted by the Brazilian Cabinet of Ministers chaired by President Jair Bolsonaro, and, in particular, by himself. They were focused both on down-

---

[13] Taking into account the value of GDP.

[14] Both taking into account the expenses measured by the current value of USD and taking into account the purchasing power parity.

[15] However, it should be remembered that Brazil is the sixth most populated country in the world.

Fig. 1. Daily number of new COVID-19 cases detected in Brazil in 2020

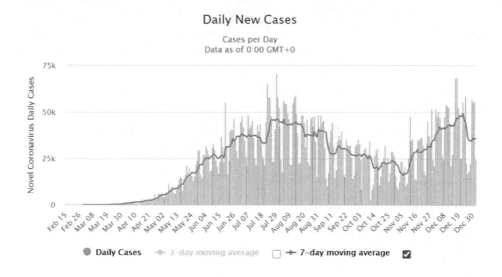

Source: Worldometers.info

Fig. 2. Daily COVID-19 deaths in Brazil in 2020

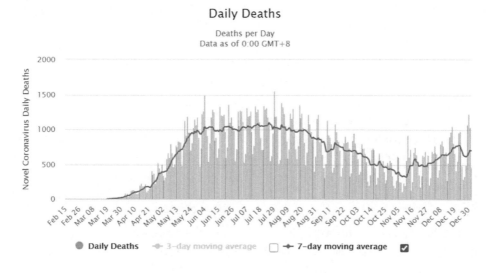

Source: Worldometers.info

playing the danger, acting against the recommendations issued by international organizations dealing with health protection and on torpedoing the initiatives of other entities aimed at controlling the epidemic. Such conduct led to the emergence of a division concerning the management of the new threat – both in the state, but also in the presidential administration.. As a result, within a month, there was a change in the position of the minister of health twice, and throughout almost the whole 2020, a clash of various forces with different priorities could be observed.

In a summary of the Brazilian federal government's strategy against the COVID-19 threat in 2020, prepared by the Research Center for Health Law (Centro De Estudos E Pesquisas De Direito Sanitario – CEPEDISA) of the University of São Paulo and the human rights organization Conectas Direitos Humanos, authors emphasize that the deaths of many people would have been prevented from prioritizing health rather than the economy. The very title of the publication is telling: *An unprecedented attack on human rights in Brazil: the timeline of the federal government's strategy to spread Covid-19.* The authors, by juxtaposing normative acts, obstructive actions, and rhetoric of the federal government, including the president himself, come to the shocking conclusion: "Our research reveals the existence of an institutional strategy promoted by the federal government, spearheaded by the Presidency of the Republic, that intentionally seeks to ensure the spread of the virus" (Ventura, Reis, 2021: 3). What particularly draws attention to the reaction of the central authorities to the threat is its depreciation and ridicule by Jair Bolsonaro. From the very beginning, the president called the virus a "fantasy" and a "measly cold", and about his fellow citizens he said that Brazilians can be immersed in sewage and "do not catch anything", and he himself, as a former athlete, has nothing to worry about, because in the event of infection "He wouldn't feel anything, or it would be just a little flu". In turn, due to the increasing number of deaths, he said, "You will all catch it someday. What are you afraid of? Face it. I'm sorry about the deaths. People die every day for many reasons. It's all part of life." At the same time, he actively began to fight restrictions and *lockdowns* introduced at the state level, calling for a return to normality, protection of jobs and the economy, and accused politicians - calling for isolation and social distance and a strong reaction of the state to the threat - of sowing panic and hysteria in order to suppress political capital. President Jair Bolsonaro actively opposed the wearing of masks, both with his attitude and by vetoing regulations imposing such an obligation. He issued decrees recognizing the activities of such enterprises as beauty and barber's salons, or gyms as crucial in the pandemic era, while at the same time torpedoing many proposals increasing economic aid for the poorest. At the same time, he promoted the use of chloroquine in case of infection, which was reflected, inter alia, in the recommendations of health ministers regarding the treatment of patients, despite the lack of clear evidence of its effectiveness (Eisenhammer, Spring, 2020; Sandy, Milhorance, 2020; Schaffner, 2020; Ventura, Reis, 2021). In this context, actions such as limiting the movement of people across borders (first with Venezuela and later also with other countries) or developing a national vaccination implementation plan seem insufficient to call them an epidemic-fighting strategy (Ventura & Reis, 2021).

Opposition to the health policy pursued by the Cabinet of Ministers under the leadership of President Jair Bolsonaro and the development of the epidemic in the country was adopted by municipal, state, and federal district authorities, as well as the National Congress and the Federal Supreme Court. These entities and their leaders, headed by the governor of the state of São Paulo, João Doria, began to work towards introducing a strategy to combat COVID-19 in line with WHO recommendations and global trends. Brazilian states began to impose restrictions on economic activity, population movement, school closures, and a lockdown. At the state level, legal provisions were also introduced, imposing social distancing and wearing masks (Andreoni, 2021; Londoño, Andreoni, Casado, 2020a; Phillips, Briso, 2020; Savarese, Biller, 2020).

Covid-19 and health policy against the epidemic in Chile

Although many reservations about the response to the outbreak of the pandemic can also be formulated against the Chilean authorities, they have adopted a different from the Brazilian approach to the fight against SARS-CoV-2, basing their risk management strategy on the recommendations of the WHO and other organizations. The country's potential to respond to the health crisis, as already mentioned, is relatively high.[16] In Chile, according to data published by the World Bank, spending on health, measured as a percentage of the state's GDP, increased from 7.03% in 2000 to 9.14% in

---

[16] Compared to other countries in the region.

2018.[17] However, taking into account the funds spent annually on health care per capita, they were the highest among South American countries and amounted to over USD 2,300[18]. However, as in the case of Brazil, the relatively good financing of the health service did not translate directly into the effectiveness of the fight against the epidemic. By December 31, more than 16.5 thousand people had died in the country as a result of COVID-19, what meant the death of 868 people per million inhabitants. Also, the number of infections per million inhabitants – nearly 32 thousand – places Chile in the lead, behind Brazil, Argentina, and Colombia (respectively: 36 thousand, 35.8 thousand, 32.1 thousand). However, what positively distinguishes Chile from the rest of the region is the high number of tests per million inhabitants – over 338,500 – almost twice as high as the second Uruguay - almost 184,000, which allows to increase the detection of infections and thus the credibility of the data on virus transmission (*Covid-19 Coronavirus Pandemic,* 2021).[19]

The first case of infection with the SARS-CoV-2 virus was recorded in Chile on March 3, and from then on, the rapid development of the epidemic in the country was noticeable, requiring government intervention. Chilean authorities, led by President Sebastián Piñera, in response to the growing threat, decided to apply the strategy recommended by the WHO (*Advice on using,* 2020). The infected persons were subjected to isolation, efforts were made to follow the route of transmission of the virus, and rules of social distancing were introduced. On March 13, a ban was introduced to organize public events of more than 500 people and a 14-day quarantine for people coming from countries with a high risk of infection was announced (*Chile bans,* 2020). On March 15, it was also decided to suspend classes in schools and universities, on March 16 to temporarily close borders, on March 18, a state of disaster was declared, and on March 22, the introduction of a night curfew was announced (Canals, Cuadrado, Canals, Yohannessen, Lefio, Bertoglia, et al., 2020; *Chile to close,* 2020). Due to the epidemic and the increasing number of infections and deaths, lockdowns were introduced in

---

[17] In 2011, they amounted to 6.77% of GDP, and, importantly, the country's GDP itself increased more than threefold in this period - from nearly USD 78 billion in 2000 to almost USD 300 billion in 2018.

[18] Taking into account the purchasing power parity. In the current value of USD, it was USD 1,455 per person, which put Chile in second place – after Uruguay, which spends USD 1,590 per person.

[19] Doubts have been raised as to the credibility of the data reported by the Chilean authorities (more: Isea, 2020; Sarwari, 2020).

Fig. 3. Daily number of new COVID-19 cases detected in Brazil in 2020

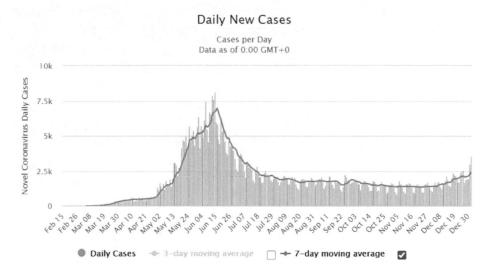

Source: Worldometers.info

Fig. 2. Daily COVID-19 deaths in Chile in 2020

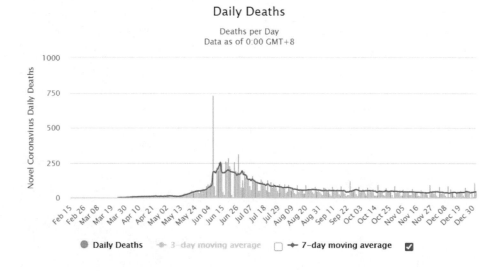

Source: Worldometers.info

individual regions of the country, including the Santiago Metropolitan Region, and from April 8, mouth and nose coverings were ordered in public transport, which was later extended to other spaces. Interestingly, even President Sebastián Piñera was fined for non-compliance of this rule (Ulloa, Castillo, 2020; *The use of masks, 2020*; Sherwood, McCool, 2020). There were also controversial issues raised in Chile regarding the introduction of the so-called immunity passport - criticized for scientific, ethical, and legal reasons - as well as frequently changed criteria and problems with recording SARS-CoV-2 infections, which led to the resignation of the Minister of Health (Bartlett, 2020; Sherwood, Ellis, 2020, Gutiérrez, 2020).

It is also worth noting that the outbreak of the SARS-CoV-2 pandemic in Chile coincided with a socio-political crisis related to mass protests by the population and the referendum on the change of the constitution planned for April 26. The restrictions introduced in response to the growing threat of the virus, including declaring a state of disaster, health alert, limiting the organization of assemblies, or assigning additional powers to the executive authorities,[20] provided the state administration with new tools also for extinguishing protests (Court, Correa, 2020). The development of the epidemic also led to the postponement of the planned referendum on the change of the constitution, which took place on October 25 (Ramos & Sherwood, 2020). In addition to efforts to reduce the spread of the virus in society by introducing restrictions, orders and prohibitions, the Chilean authorities also focused on supporting the economy. A stimulating financial package was launched at the level of 4.7% of the state's GDP – nearly USD 12 billion, aimed to protect jobs and support small and medium-sized enterprises, tax breaks and benefits for employees were introduced, employment regulations were made more flexible, and the Central Bank had lowered interest rates (more: Lyon, Martinez, Cuevaz, 2020).

Summary

The spread of the Covid-19 epidemic in South America has been and continues to be a serious challenge for the countries of the region. Their actions

---

[20] For example, undersecretaries in the ministry of health obtained the right to set maximum prices for pharmaceutical and medical products, health products and services, and to regulate their sale (*Modifica Decreto* N° 4, 2020: Art.:1; Court, Correa, 2020)

had both unilateral and multilateral dimensions, and the strategies adopted were often extremely different, as evidenced by the responses to the threat from Brazil and Chile.

In the first country, the federal government, led by the president, decided to downplay, ignore and put economic issues before the health and safety of citizens. As a result, this has led to Brazil being indicating as an example of not coping with the crisis, which has tragic consequences in the form of the death of thousands of people. The reported data – on new infections and deaths – shows that in the case of this country, it is difficult to talk about controlling or stabilizing the situation, and the emerging trends cannot be said to be optimistic. It is therefore not surprising that the country has built up internal opposition to the Jair Bolsonaro administration, which has taken alternative measures to contain the spread of the virus.

Most countries in the region followed a different path than the Brazilian one, taking actions recommended by WHO and other organizations. In Chile, the focus was on limiting direct social interactions, introducing a partial *lockdown*, introducing distancing, covering the mouth, and social isolation. The actions taken were reflected in the statistics on the development of the epidemic. On their basis, it can be concluded that they contributed to the stabilization of the situation, and the prospect of the virus spreading, also taking into account the implementation of vaccinations, allows us to look to the future with hope.

The response to the spread of SARS-CoV-2 in South America was also of a transnational nature. The countries of the region, within the framework of the existing organizations, began to provide information on the dynamics of the epidemic development and the actions taken by them, and also launched additional mechanisms, including financial and training, to support decision-making processes and strategies undertaken by individual countries. They also declared joint purchases on the market of medical and pharmaceutical products under PROSUR. These activities demonstrate the readiness of states to strengthen cooperation and at the same time increase their ability to respond to the epidemic threat, but it should also be remembered that earlier integration initiatives - such as UNASUR, which could have a really high potential to fight COVID-19 – were due to ideological reasons discontinued or replaced with new ones. Perhaps the pandemic will be a turning point in the processes of tightening ties in the region, showing the rulers the need to coordinate policies and the advantages of cooperation, resulting, for example, from synergies and economies of scale.

References

14-day COVID-19 case notification rate per 100 000, weeks 52–53 (2021), "European Center for Disease Prevention and Control", https://www.ecdc.europa.eu/en/geographical-distribution-2019 -ncov-cases, (Accessed: 07/01/2021).

Acuerdo de Integracion Subregional Andino (Acuerdo de Cartagena) (1969), "Comunidad Andina", http://www.comunidadandina.org/Documentos.aspx, (Accessed: 13.01.2021).

Advice on the use of masks in the community, during home care and in health care settings in the context of the novel coronavirus (2019-nCoV) outbreak (2020), WHO, https://apps.who.int/iris/bitstream /handle/10665/330987/WHO-nCov-IPC_Masks-2020.1-eng.pdf?sequence=1&isAllowed=y, (Accessed: 13.01.2021).

Andreoni M. (2021) *Coronavirus in Brazil: What You Need to Know*, "The New York Times", https://www.nytimes.com/article/brazil-coronavirus-cases.html, (Accessed: 13.01.2021).

Aneiros Fernandez et. al. (2013), *Salud Pública en MERCOSUR*,"Escuela Andaluza de Salud Pública", https://www.easp.es/?wpdmact=process&did=MTIyLmhvdGxpbms=, (Accessed: 13.01.2021).

Bartlett J. (2020), *Chile's health minister quits over government response to Covid-19*,"The Guardian", https://www.theguardian.com/global-development/2020/jun/14/chiles-health-minister-   quits-over-government-response-to-covid-19, (Accessed: 13.01.2021).

Canals M, Cuadrado C, Canals A, Yohannessen K, Lefio LA, Bertoglia MP, et al. (2020), *Epidemic trends, public health response and health system capacity: the Chilean experience in four months of the COVID-19 pandemic*, "Rev Panam Salud Publica" vol. 44, DOI: https://doi.org/10.26633/RPSP.2020.99.

Chile bans large public events over coronavirus fears, ahead of planned protests (2020), "Reuters", https://www.reuters.com/article/us-health-coronavirus-chile-idUSKBN21102N, (Accessed: 7.01.2021).

Chile to close borders to foreign travelers beginning Wednesday (2020), "Reuters", https://www.reuters.com/article/us-chile-coronavirus-idUSKBN213289,   (Accessed: 13.01.2021).

Constitution of the Pan American Sanitary Organization (1947), Pan American Sanitary Organization Meeting Of The Directing Council, Buenos Aires, September 24, 1947OSP / DC / A / 16 (corrected), "Pan American Health Organization", https: // iris.paho.org / bitstream / handle / 10665.2 / 25925 / a192777.pdf? sequence = 1 & isAllowed = y, (Accessed: 01.09.2021).

Coronavirus Disease (COVID-19) pandemic (2021), "Pan American Health Organization", https://www.paho.org/en/topics/coronavirus-infections/coronavirus-disease-covid-19-pandemic, (Accessed: 01/13/2021).

Court J., Correa JT (2020), *Chile's Political and Institutional Response to COVID-19,* "The Regulatory Review", https://www.theregreview.org/2020/06/24/court-correa-chile-political- institutional-response-covid-19 / (Accessed: 7.01.2021).

COVD-19 - PAHO / WHO Response. 07 December 2020. Report 37 (2020), "Pan American Health Organization", https://www.paho.org/en/documents/covid-19-pahowho-response-report-37–07-december-2020, (Accessed: 13.01. 2021).

COVID-19 ¿Que es y cómo prevenirlo (2021), "El Organismo Andino de Salud - Convenio Hipólito Unanue", http://orasconhu.org/portal/node/596, (Accessed: 13.01.2021).

Covid-19 Coronavirus Pandemic (2021), "Worldometer", https://www.worldometers.info/coronavirus/, (Accessed: 01.01.2021).

De Lima L., Bruera E. (2000), *The Pan American Health Organization: Its Structure and Role in the Development of a Palliative Care Program for Latin America and the Caribbean,* "Journal of Pain and Symptom Management", Vol. 20, No. December 6, 2000.

De Sousa M. Savarese M. (2020), *Brazil confirms first coronavirus case in Latin America,* "Associated Press News", https://apnews.com/article/fd3d0d0120dd-10f3d09bad78a4dd9539, (Accessed: 07.01.2021).

Decision 445, Adscripción del Convenio Hipólito Unanue al Sistema Andino de Integración (1998), "Gaceta Oficial del Acuerdo de Cartagena", Año XV - Número 364, http://intranet.comunidadandina Decision.org/Documentos/gacetas/gace364.PDF, (Accessed: 13.01.2021).

Declaracion de los presidentes del mercosur sobre coordinacion regional para la contencion y mitigacion del coronavirus y su impacto (2020), "Mercado Común del Sur", https://documentos.mercosur.int/simfiles/declaraciones/Declaracio%CC%81n% 20COVID-19.pdf, (Accessed: 13.01.2021).

Della Coletta R. (2020), Bolsonaro *Criticizes The Closure of Schools, Attacks Governors and Blames the Media in Televised Statement,* "Folha de S. Paulo", https://www1.folha.uol.com.br/internacional/en /brazil/2020/03/bolsonaro-criticizes-the-closure-of-schools-attacks-governors-and-blames-the-media-in-televised-statement.shtml, (Accessed: 13.01.2021).

Eisenhammer S., Spring J. (2020), *Bolsonaro urges Brazilians back to work, dismisses coronavirus 'hysteria',* "Reuters", https://www.reuters.com/article/us-health-coronavirus-brazil/bolsonaro- urges-brazilians-back-to-work-dismisses-coronavirus-hysteria-idUSKBN21B2H2, (Accessed: 13.01.2021).

Epstein D., Nusser N. (2021), *PAHO raises $ 263 million in 2020 to fight COVID-19 in the Americas,* "Pan American Health Organization", https://www.paho.org/en/news/12–1 -2021-paho-raises-263-million-2020-fight-covid-19-americas, (Accessed: 13.01.2021).

Gutiérrez I. (2020), *El pasaporte de inmunidad, un experimento descartado en todo el mundo que ya hizo rectificar al gobierno de Chile,* "El Diario", https://www.eldiario.es/internacional/pasaporte-inmunidad-experimento -descartado-mundo-hizo-rectificar-gobierno-chile_1_6132598.html, (Accessed: 13.01.2021).

Herraro MB, Tussie D. (2015), *UNASUR Health: A quiet revolution in health diplomacy in South America*, "Global Social Policy", Vol. 15 (3), DOI: https://doi.org/10.1177/1468018115599818.

Informe de Gestión PROSUR 2019–2020 (2020), "Foro para el Progreso de América del Sur (PROSUR)", https://foroprosur.org/wp-content/uploads/2020/12/PROSUR_Informe_de_Gestion_2020.pdf, (Accessed: 13.01.2021).

Isea R. (2020), *How Valid are the Reported Cases of People Infected with Covid-19 in the World?*, "International Journal Of Coronaviruses", Vol-1 Issue 2., DOI: 10.14302 / issn.2692–1537.ijcv-20–3376.

Londoño E., Andreoni M., Casado L. (2020a), *Brazil, Once a Leader, Struggles to Contain Virus Amid Political Turmoil, "The New York Times", https://www.nytimes.com/2020/05/ 16 /world / americas / virus-brazil-deaths.html, (Accessed: 13.01.2021).

Londoño E., Andreoni M., Casado L. (2020b), Bolsonaro, *Isolated and Defiant, Dismisses Coronavirus Threat to Brazil,* "The New York Times", https://www.nytimes.com/2020/04/01/ world / americas / brazil-bolsonaro-coronavirus.html, (Accessed: 13.01.2021).

Lyon F., Martinez A., Cuevaz A. (2020), *Chile: Government and institution measures in response to COVID-19,* "KPMG", https://home.kpmg/xx/en/home/insights/2020/ 04 / chile-government-and-institution-measures-in-response-to-covid.html, (Accessed: 07.01.2021).

Mausoleum of broken institutions (2019), "The Economist", March 23rd, 2019.

Modifica Decreto N° 4, de 2020, del Ministerio de Salud, que Decreta Alerta Sanitaria por el Período que Se Señala y Otorga Facultades Extraordinarias que Indica por Emergencia de Salud Pública de Importancia Internacional (Espii) por Brote del Nuevo Coronavirus (2019-Ncov), Núm. 10. Santiago, 24 de Marzo de 2020, Normas Generales CVE 1745010, Diario Oficial de la Republica de Chile, Núm. 42.614, Miércoles 25 de Marzo de 2020.

Moll AA (1941), *The Pan American Sanitary Bureau: Its origin, development and achievements*, "Boletin de la Oficina Sanitaria Panamericana", Afio 20, No. 1, "Pan American Health Organization", https://iris.paho.org/bitstream/handle/10665.2/13954/v20n1p41.pdf?sequence=1&isAllowed=y, (Accessed: 09.01.2021).

Phillips T., Briso CB (2020), *Bolsonaro 's anti-science response to coronavirus appals Brazil's governors,*"The Guardian", https://www.theguardian.com/world/2020/mar/27/jair-bolsonaro-coronavirus- brazil-governors-appalled, (Accessed: 13.01.2021).

Ramos N., Sherwood D. (2020), *Chile to postpone referendum on new constitution as coronavirus concerns grow,* "Reuters", https://www.reuters.com/article/us-health-coronavirus-chile/chile-to -postpone-referendum-on-new-constitution-as-coronavirus-concerns-grow-idUSKBN2163TL, (Accessed: 07.01.2021).

Rodriguez-Morales AJ, Gallego V, Escalera-Antezana JP, Mendez CA et. al., (2020), *COVID-19 in Latin America: The implications of the first confirmed case in Brazil,* "Travel Medicine and Infectious Disease", Vol. 35, May – June 2020, DOI: https://doi.org/10.1016/j.tmaid.2020.101613.

Salud (2021), "Mercado Común del Sur", https://www.mercosur.int/temas/salud/, (Accessed: 13.01.2021).

Sandy M., Milhorance F. (2020), *Brazil's President Still Insists the Coronavirus Is Overblown. These Governors Are Fighting Back,* "Time", https://time.com/5816243/brazil-jair-bolsonaro-coronavirus-governors/, (Accessed: 13.01.2021).

Sarwari K. (2020), *A pandemic lesson from Chile: data transparency can save lives,* "News @ Northeastern", https://news.northeastern.edu/2020/08/17/a-pandemic-lesson-from-chile -data-transparency-plays-a-key-role-in-saving-lives /, (Accessed: 13.01.2021).

Savarese M., Biller D. (2020), *Brazil's governors rise up against Bolsonaro's virus stance,* "The Associated Press", https://apnews.com/article/36fa0e82581a1fdd6b97f2c34ccc9b1d, (Accessed: 13.01.2021).

Schaffner F. (2020), *Inaugurações, aglomerações e cloroquina: como foi a visita de Bolsonaro a Bagé,* "GZH Portal", https://gauchazh.clicrbs.com.br/politica/noticia/2020/07/inauguracoes-aglomeracoes -e cloroquina-como-foi-a-visita-de-bolsonaro-a-bage-ckdanu88b0043013gksm8zb3d.html, (Accessed: 13.01.2021).

Sherwood D., Ellis A. (2020), *In reversal, Chile says coronavirus release certificates will not prove immunity,* "Reuters", https://www.reuters.com/article/us-health-coronavirus-chile-idUSKBN22B2ZY, (Accessed: 13.01.2021).

Sherwood D., McCool G. (2020), *Chilean president handed $ 3,500 fine for maskless selfie with stranger on beach,* "Reuters", https://www.reuters.com/article/us-chile-coronavirus-idUSKBN213289, (Accessed: 13.01.2021).

Specialized Organizations (2021), "The Organization of American States", http://www.oas.org/en/about/specialized_organizations.asp, (Accessed: 01.09.2021).

Technical Documents - Coronavirus Disease (COVID-19) (2021), "Pan American Health Organization", https://www.paho.org/en/technical-documents-coronavirus-disease-covid-19, (Accessed: 13.01. 2021).

The PAHO COVID-19 Response Fund (2021), "Pan American Health Organization", https://www.paho.org/en/topics/coronavirus-infections/coronavirus-disease-covid-19-pandemic/paho-covid- 19-response-fund, (Accessed: 13.01.2021).

The use of masks in enclosed public spaces becomes mandatory (2020), "Chile reports", https://chilereports.cl/en/news/2020/04/20/the-use-of-masks-in-enclosed-public -spaces-becomes-mandatory, (Accessed: 13.01.2021).

The World Bank (2021), https://data.worldbank.org/, (Accessed: 13.01.2021).

Tratado Constitutivo de la Unión de Naciones Suramericanas (2008), "Universidad Nacional de la Plata", http://sedici.unlp.edu.ar/bitstream/handle/10915/45568/ UNASUR_-_Tratado_Constitutivo_de_la_Uni%C3ac%C3nSur_de_la_ Uni%C3ac%C3nSur._.pdf? sequence = 3, (Accessed: 13.01.2021).

Ulloa C., Castillo J. (2020), *Chile mandates face masks on public and private transportation,* "CNN", https://edition.cnn.com/world/live-news/coronavirus-pandemic-04–07–20 / h_ea210ada6a6ce92232c0a062bc83af11, (Accessed: 13.01.2021).

Ventura, D., Reis, R. (2021), *An unprecedented attack on human rights in Brazil: the timeline of the federal government's strategy to spread Covid-19,* Offprint, trans. Luis Misiara, "Bulletin Rights in the Pandemic" No. 10, São Paulo, Brazil, CEPEDISA / USP and Conectas Human Rights., Https://www.conectas.org/ wp/wp-content/uploads/2021/01/10boletimcovid_english_03.pdf, (Accessed: 03.02.2021).

Piotr Baranowski
Uniwersytet im. Adama Mickiewicza w Poznaniu
ORCID: 0000-0002-9598-7463
Maria Spychała-Kij
Uniwersytet im. Adama Mickiewicza w Poznaniu
ORCID: 0000-0001-6793-9440

SARS-COV-2 IN THE ARAB WORLD - CONDITIONS OF SPREADING, PREVENTION, AND TACKLING THE PANDEMIC[1]

The following work aims to describe the development of the pandemic, caused by SARS-COVID-2 virus, in the Arab World. A multifactoral comparative analysis with the use of basic methods of data analysis is aimed at showing the correlation between selected social and economic indicators of the countries included in the Arab World and the number of infections, mortality rate, and the rate of infection and recovery growth. The analysis carried out in this way will allow for a preliminary assessment of the effectiveness of the preventive and intervention measures taken in the selected geographic area. In May of 2020, the authors delivered a speech at the 1st International e-Conference "The world in the age of pandemic and post-pandemic period" organized at the Faculty of Political Science and Journalism of the Adam Mickiewicz University, in which they posed a hypothesis that the high number of infections recorded among the richest countries of the Arab World, is likely to be related to the wealth of these countries, which further translates into a high level of expenditure on health care, which translates into the number of tests being performed as higher than that in the other countries in the region. In May 2020, there was not yet enough data to con-

---

[1] The research was financed from the project „Research on COVID-19" from the funds of the Adam Mickiewicz University , Poznan

firm said hypothesis, although there were indications that it was accurate. However, in September this year, convincing data emerged that show that the initial assumptions were true. The data used for this analysis come from publicly available sources, such as the World Bank, the International Monetary Fund, specialized UN agencies, the CIA Factbook[2] and regional media reports publishing information in English.

The Arab World is a rather peculiar category within the field of political science research, mainly due to the fact, that the main criterion distinguishing this geographic and social entity, is the membership of states in the largest international organization within the region - the League of Arab States. The Arab World comprises the territory of the Middle East, North Africa (MENA), and part of East Africa. Currently, there are 22 member states of the Arab League: Algeria, Saudi Arabia, Bahrain, Djibouti, Egypt, Iraq, Yemen, Jordan, Qatar, Comoros, Kuwait, Lebanon, Libya, Morocco, Mauritania, Oman, Palestine, Somalia, Sudan, Syria, Tunisia and the United Arab Emirates (UAE). Membership of the Syrian Republic has been suspended since 2011. In 2017, the GDP of all the member states of the LAS (2,513 trillion USD) (*Arab World GDP*, World Bank 2020) was almost six times lower than the GDP of the European Union (14 736 trillion USD) (*UE GDP*, World Bank 2020) and almost equal to India's GDP (2,653 trillion USD) (*India GDP*, World Bank 2020) at the same time accounting for only 3% of the global GDP (81,229 trillion USD) (*World GDP*, World Bank 2020). Among the League countries, Saudi Arabia has the highest GDP (792,967 billion in 2019) while the lowest Comoros (1,186 billion in 2019) (*Saudi Arabia, Comoros GDP*, World Bank 2020). In 2019 the population of the Arab World amounted to 427,870 million, which accounts for only 5% of the global population (*Population total*, World Bank 2020), which shows that the economy of these states is much below the optimal level, accounting for only 3% of the global GDP.

Human Development Index and healthcare expenditure

Out of all the states of the Arab World, only 6 could boast in having scored over 0,8 on the HDI index and all of them were the rich monarchies of the

---

[2] Appendix CIA FactBook in the bibliography.

Arabian Peninsula. UAE (0,866), Saudi Arabia (0,857), Qatar (0,848), Bahrain (0,838), Oman (0,834) and Kuwait (0,808) (*UNDP, HDI Report 2019*). The lowest scores were recorded in the peripheral poor republics with a high level of corruption or, as in the case of Yemen and Syria, countries affected by a humanitarian crisis resulting from an armed conflict. Somalia (0,285), Djibouti (0,495), Yemen (0,463), Sudan (0,507), Mauritania (0,527), Comoros (0,54) and Syria (0,549) had an HDI below 6 according to data for 2019 (*UNDP, HDI Report 2019*).

One of the components of the HDI index is life expectancy, which to a large extent depends on the quality of the health care system. Spending on healthcare closely corresponds to the HDI, however, only when the expenditure per capita is taken into account. When absolute values are considered, Egypt and Iraq spend much more than Bahrain or Kuwait, but when taking into account the number of inhabitants of these countries, it turns out that the highest per capita spending can be observed among the five wealthy monarchies of the Arabian Peninsula, yet this time without the inclusion of Oman, which falls behind Lebanon. The below values denote the sum in USD per person in 2017: Qatar (1649), Kuwait (1509), UAE (1310), Bahrain (1127), Saudi Arabia (1093); countries with the lowest HDI index were ranked lowest, namely Yemen (70,3), Djibouti (70,3), Comoros (58,7), Mauritania (48,8) and Syria (68,8). The average for the Arab World in 2017 totaled 245,79 USD. (*Current Health Expenditure*, World Bank 2020).

Dates of the first detected cases

The SARS-COVID-2 virus has reached the Arab World from various locations. Despite the knowledge regarding the first detected case in each of the LAS countries and the knowledge of the place from which the virus was imported, it is almost certain that they were not the actual initial cases. The first country to report the presence of the virus was the United Arab Emirates, which happened on January 30, 2020, in a person arriving from the People's Republic of China. According to the obtained knowledge, the virus last arrived in the Comoros, where the first case was recorded on May 1, 2020. (*Comoros confirms*, 2020). The below table shows the sequence in which the first case of the virus was detected in different member states.

Healthcare expenditure per capita and order of first case detection

Countries with the highest expenditure on health care per capita, according to the previously presented data are Qatar, Kuwait, UAE, Bahrain, Saudi Arabia, followed by Lebanon, Oman, Iraq, and Egypt. In light of these figures and of the compiled order in which the first infections were detected among the LAS member states (Figure 1), a correlation is visible. All the above-mentioned countries that spend the most on health services per capita are at the same time those countries where the infection occurred most quickly, or where there were an effective detection and a record of the first case.

Figure 1. Health expenditure per capita in USD

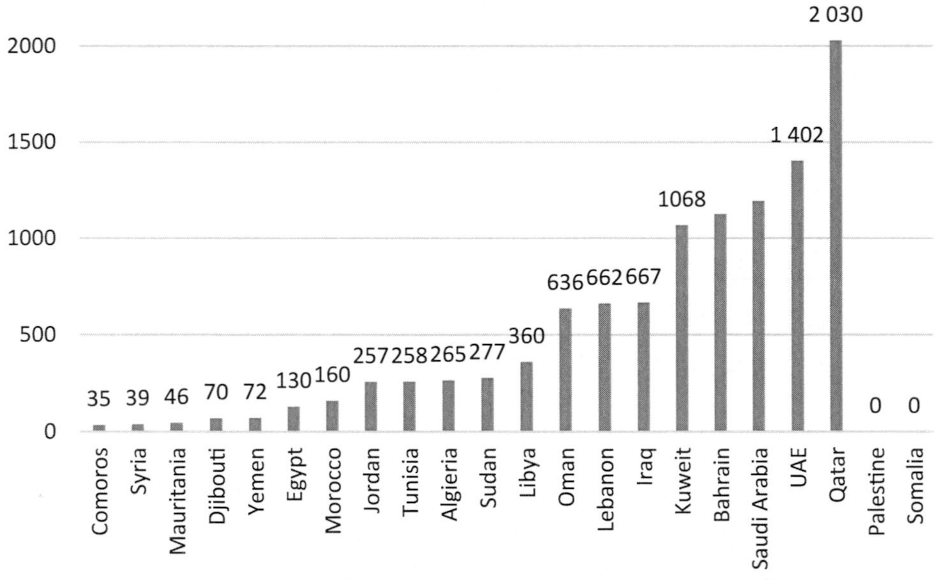

S o u r c e: *World Bank, Current health expenditure per capita (current US$) - Saudi Arabia, Qatar, Syrian Arab Republic, Comoros, Yemen, Rep., Iraq, Libya, Djibouti, Somalia, Bahrain, Sudan, Mauritania, Jordan, Lebanon, Kuwait, Morocco, Tunisia, Oman, Egypt, Arab Rep., Algeria, United Arab Emirates, https://data.worldbank.org/indicator/SH.XPD.CHEX. PC.CD?locations=SA-QA-SY-KM-YE-IQ-LY-DJ-SO-BH-SD-MR-JO-LB-KW-MA-TN-OM-EG-DZ-AE, (Accessed: 17/05/2020).;*

Source of the first detected case[3]

The virus was brought in from various locations. Based on the first detected cases, it can be concluded that the two sources of the outbreak of infection from which the virus was transferred to the LPA countries are Iran and the People's Republic of China. In the light of the information on the first detected case, it appears that the virus was imported from Iran to Iraq, Lebanon, Kuwait, Saudi Arabia, Qatar, Bahrain, and Oman and that it was spread from China to the United Arab Emirates, Somalia, and Egypt, and from Italy, it was passed on to Syria, Tunisia, and Morocco, from Spain to Djibouti, from Greece to Palestine and from France to Mauritania. To Sudan, it was transferred from the UAE.

It can be observed that despite the time intervals between the dates of the first detected case in the individual LPA states, the first transmission of the virus did not take place as a result of contact with another previously infected LPA country, but rather was imported from the countries outside of the region. The exception is the aforementioned Libya and Sudan, to which the virus came respectively from Saudi Arabia and the UAE. This suggests that in the initial stage of spreading the virus among LAS countries, geographical proximity was not the most important factor as no domino effect could be observed. It appears that air connectivity and the level of globalization of the specific country played a more important role than land connection. This explains the two exceptions already mentioned, in which Saudi Arabia and the UAE were sources of infection. It is, however, still surprising that there appears to have been so little virus exchange between LPA countries in terms of the first recorded case, in light of the fact that for 2014 data the United Arab Emirates, or more specifically Dubai, is the sixth largest airport in terms of traffic, and even the first when only international flights are considered (*Airport Traffic Ranking, Airports Council International,* 2014) and Saudi Arabia respectively also hosts Muslims from all over the world due to its religious sites.

---

[3] Appendix 1.

Analysis of infection statistics in LAS countries

By May 1, 2020, the virus had reached all 22 states of the Arab League. As of May 17, the absolute number of infections was highest in Saudi Arabia with 54,752 detected cases and lowest in the Comoros, where 11 infections were recorded. By that date, as many as 5 out of 22 countries had recorded more than 10,000 cases. Those being: Saudi Arabia (54,752), Qatar (30,972), UAE (23,358), Kuwait (14,850) and Egypt (12,229)[4]. At the same time, those are also countries in which the virus was detected relatively early: UAE as the first, Egypt as the second, Kuwait as the sixth, Qatar as the seventh, and Saudi Arabia as the eighth country in the region. Despite the relative dependence, it is impossible to claim a direct correlation between the number of infections and the date of detection of the first case. Presented below is a table with the number of detected cases as of May 17, 2020.

Figure 2. The total number of cases in the Arab World on 17th of May 2020

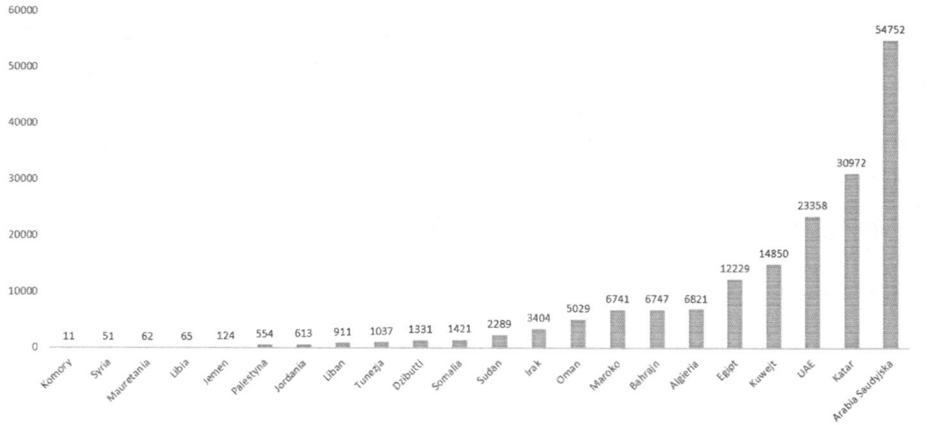

S o u r c e: Worldometers info (https://www.worldometers.info/coronavirus/#countries, accessed 17/05/2020).

When it comes to the increase in infections, the number of infections increased the fastest where the number of detected infections is currently (as of May 17, 2020) the highest. The table below presents data on the rate of increase in infections, obtained by dividing the absolute number of infections by the number of days from the first detected infection to May 17, 2020.

---

[4] Appendix 1

There may be several reasons explaining why on average there were more infections detected in some places than in others. Initially, it was checked whether there is a possible relation between the increase in the number of infections and the population density in a given area. While it is difficult to talk about a direct correlation between population density and the average daily increase in infection for all countries, it is noticeable in the case of the UAE, Kuwait, and Qatar. However, no correlation was observed in the case of Saudi Arabia, therefore, the hypothesis could not be confirmed.

Further, it was checked whether the increase of detected cases was related to the speed of introducing the first restrictions aimed at preventing infections or slowing down their increase. For this purpose, the numbers of detected cases were arranged in the order in which the first restrictions were introduced in a given country. The results show that only in the case of some of the countries their delayed reaction could be linked to a bigger number of infections; that is mainly the case of Kuwait (9 days after the first case detected), Qatar (11 days after the first case detected), Egypt (31 days after the first case detected) and UAE (39 days from the first detected case). The relationship between the two indicators is, however, by no means apparent. Saudi Arabia constitutes an interesting case, where despite the introduction of restrictions up to 25 days before the first infection was detected, the increase and the total number of infections remain the highest. In addition to preventive or remedial measures, several countries have implemented changes aimed at improving the economic situation. For example, the level of compulsory bank reserves was reduced to maintain financial liquidity, which was observed in the wealthy monarchies of the Persian Gulf (*Policy Responses to COVID-19*, 2020).

Despite the demonstrated lack of a clear relationship between the speed of the introduction of the first restrictions and the number of incoming cases, there is a clear correlation between the speed and the form of the first action taken. In eight countries, restrictions were implemented even before the first infection occurred. Those countries are Saudi Arabia, Iraq, Djibouti, Syria, Yemen, Libya, Comoros, Somalia, and among them, the majority introduced border restrictions as the first action, except for Iraq, where a curfew was introduced instead, and Somalia, which closed schools. It is important to highlight the peculiar and unstable political situation present in most of these countries, which could have influenced both the decision on the type of action taken as well as the accuracy of the available data. An interesting correlation appears when we divide the given countries according to their political system. Seven of the LAS countries have closed their borders as their first action and all of them, except for Saudi Arabia, are republics. All the monarchies (except for aforementioned Saudi Arabia) delayed their restrictions and in the first step did not attempt to close the borders but rather introduced restrictions in schools and/or places of worship. The reason for such a correlation may be that the LAS monarchies are also all those countries with the highest GDP in the region, i.e. UAE, Oman, Kuwait, Qatar, Bahrain, Saudi Arabia, except for Morocco and Jordan with a comparably average GDP level. This suggests that the economic interests, the degree of development, and globalization of a given country may have influenced the type of the first action that the said state decided on implementing.

A conclusion may be reached, that implementation of border restrictions was a measure enforced in states that acted in a preventive manner. On the other hand, after the first infection was already detected, the borders were closed only by the republics; monarchies (except Saudi Arabia) did not act preventively, thus they did not close the borders in the first place, but rather decided on other restrictions, such as the closure of schools and places of worship.

It is only after comparing cases of infection with health expenditure per capita that a certain relationship can be noticed. It appears that the countries that spend the most on the healthcare system per capita are also the countries with the highest number of cases.

Figure 3. Average growth and health expenditure per capita

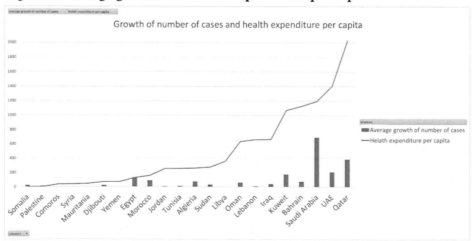

S o u r c e: Worldometers info (https://www.worldometers.info/coronavirus/#countries, accessed: 17/05/2020)

When presenting this information in mid-May 2020, it was suspected that the number of detected infections depends primarily on expenditure on health care per capita and thus on potentially more tests being carried out. In the table above, countries such as Egypt and Algeria have relatively low spending with relatively high rates of infection. Therefore, there are two possible scenarios: either the number of cases detected in these countries is proportionately too low than in reality and it is due to not enough testing being done, or Egypt and Algeria have the best health services in the entire Arab World.

An attempt was made to test the second hypothesis by comparing the infant mortality rate to health expenditure per capita. Such comparison showed the probability of the health services in Egypt and Algeria not being as high as the number of detected cases would indicate. Figure 6 shows that infant mortality is inversely proportional to health expenditure per capita in the Arab World. This suggests that there are potentially many more cases in Algeria and Egypt than the number reported right now, but there is simply not enough testing being done. Similarly, it is likely to apply also in the case of the wealthy monarchies in the Arabian Peninsula, whose numbers appear to be more compelling.

Table 1. The number of tests per thousand and GDP per capita

Country		Total tests per thousand	GDP per capita international-$
United Arab Emirates		Sep 8 ● 778.97	$67,293
Bahrain		Sep 8 ● 702.24	$43,291
Luxembourg		Sep 7 ● 636.42	$94,278
Denmark		Sep 7 ● 466.07	$46,683
Malta		Sep 6 ● 461.48	$36,513
United States		Sep 6 ● 281.87	$54,225
Iceland		Sep 7 ● 274.57	$46,483
Russia		Sep 8 ● 269.23	$24,766
Australia		Sep 8 ● 263.94	$44,649
United States, units unclear (incl. non-PCR)		Sep 8 ● 251.84	
Lithuania		248.54	$29,524
Qatar		Sep 6 ● 231.84	$116,936
Maldives		Sep 7 ● 225.97	$15,184
Belgium		Sep 7 ● 212.74	$42,659
Portugal		Sep 6 ● 211.21	$27,937
Ireland		Sep 8 ● 184.93	$67,335
New Zealand		Sep 8 ● 172.43	$36,086
Belarus		Sep 7 ● 168.40	$17,168
Saudi Arabia		Sep 8 ● 157.95	$49,045
Canada		156.09	$44,018
Italy, tests performed		Sep 8 ● 154.88	
Kuwait		Sep 7 ● 151.75	$65,531
Norway		Sep 7 ● 147.05	$64,800
Serbia		Sep 6 ● 145.95	$14,049
Latvia		Sep 8 ● 141.93	$25,064
Austria		Sep 8 ● 141.73	$45,437
Chile		Sep 8 ● 139.65	$22,767

S o u r c e: Our World in Data, Oxford University (Number of Test per country, Our World in Data, Oxford 2020, accessed 10/09/2020)

It wasn't until September 2020 that it was possible to find evidence that potentially confirmed the previously posed hypothesis about the number of tests performed. On September 9, the Oxford University statistics portal Our World in Data published an estimate of the number of tests performed per 1,000 inhabitants and correlated them with GDP per capita in countries around the world. It showed that the countries performing the most tests in the Arab World are UAE, Bahrain, Qatar, Saudi Arabia, and Kuwait. Although, in a different order, the same countries had the highest number of detected infections in the Arab World as of May 17, when the hypothesis was posed.

Analysis of recovery and death statistics

As of May 17, when most of the data regarding recoveries and deaths was collected, different countries appeared at the top of the table than when it comes to the number of infections detected. To obtain an average recovery rate, the number of infected people that went through recovery was divided by the overall number of infections. It turned out that Tunisia performed best (77.82% of recoveries), followed by Djibouti (73.03%), then Syria (70.59%), then Iraq (67.86%), Jordan (67.37%), Morocco (55.75%), Libya (53.85%), Algeria (49.98%) and only Saudi Arabia, Bahrain, UAE, Oman, Kuwait, Lebanon, Comoros, Egypt, Qatar, Mauritania, Somalia, Sudan, Palestine, and Yemen. However, the presented data are not reliable. The first three countries (Tunisia, Djibouti, and Syria) had the number of detected infections below 1500 (Syria only 51 sic!), In Jordan only 613, and in Libya 65. It is clear, that this is too small a sample for the data to be compared with the tens of thousands of infections that appear in the countries with the highest levels of infection.

Therefore, if we exclude from the overview the countries with a relatively low number of infections, it appears that the best ratio of recoveries to infections is in Iraq (67.86% with 3,404 infections), Morocco (55.75% with 6,741 infections), Algeria (49.98% with 6,821 infections), Saudi Arabia (47.07% with 54,752 infections), Bahrain (40.80% with 6,747 infections), UAE (36.44% with 23,358 infections), Oman (29.75% with 5,029 infections), Kuwait (29.22% with 14,850 infections), Egypt (25.94% with 12,229 infections) and Qatar (15.82% with 30,972 infections). At the very bottom of the list are Mauritania, Somalia, Sudan, Palestine, and Yemen, however, they are not taken into account because of their absolute number of cases being relatively low (which, *nota bene*, should be even more alarming given the political situation in these countries).

When it comes to the number of deaths, as of May 17, 2020, the number is not particularly high, although it can be expected to increase. After placing the countries in order in terms of the number of deaths, it turns out that the following countries are in the lead: Egypt (630), Algeria (542), Saudi Arabia (312), UAE (220), Morocco (192), Iraq (127) and Kuwait (118). States, where the number of deaths was below 20, are also those countries with the lowest number of detected cases, although there are exceptions here as well: Yemen, despite only 124 cases, recorded as many as 19 deaths (mortality 15%).

Case Study: Saudi Arabia

Kingdom of Saudi Arabia despite not being the largest population-wise within the Arab World had recorded the highest number of COVID-19 among all members of the Arab League reaching 364 929 cases as of 3rd of January 2021 (*COVID-19 in Saudi Arabia*, 2020). Fortunately though thanks to the countries well-funded healthcare system, it enjoyed one of the highest rates of recovery as well, with well over 357 000 recoveries (*Saudi Arabia Ministry of Helath*, 2020). Saudi Arabia remains a leader of the Arab World in terms of the number of tests performed daily, as well as in the number of recoveries from COVID-19. In terms of testing, as of January 2021, the Kingdom's rate of positive tests among all the tests performed is 0,4%, which is one of the best rates in the world (*Saudi Arabia COVID-19 testing*, 2020). During 2020 number of tests per 1000 was sharply increasing up to the mid-August and then steadily declined (on the 15 of August it was 1,93 tests per 1000, on January 19th it was 1,38). As of January 20th, the Kingdom did not see the second wave of infections observable in countries like Egypt or UAE.

KSA was one of the earliest responders to the threat of pandemic spread in the Arab World, introducing the first domestic precautionary restrictions 24 days before the first case was identified on the 3rd of March 2020 (*Saudi Arabia Identifies*, 2020). Despite WHO's numerous calls not to restrict any commercial, political, or civil relations with China, authorities of KSA banned flights to and from China on the 6th of February 2020. Just as for most neighboring countries (Iraq, Syria, Kuwait, Bahrain, Qatar, and Oman) first reported case in Saudi Arabia was a person traveling from Iran. In com-

Figure 4. Daily New Cases in Saudi Arabia

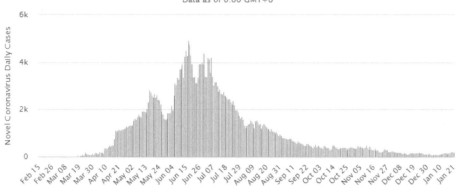

S o u r c e: Worldometer https://www.worldometers.info/coronavirus/country/saudi-arabia/ (Accessed: 22/01/2021.

parison to the rest of the Arab World, especially the republics, KSA handled the pandemic exceptionally well, as the number of new cases peaked in mid-June 2020 and started to steadily decline until it reached under 200 new cases a day at the beginning of December 2020.

Decisive actions taken at the beginning of February did not stop the spread of the virus, but it may have contributed to curbing it later on. On the 5th of February, authorities banned Umrah pilgrimage and introduced the first restrictions in terms of worship (*Saudi Arabia closes Grand Mosque*, 2020). That ban will be periodically lifted and reintroduced, according to the number of cases throughout 2020. The same month Saudi Arabia suspended entry to the holy cities of Mecca and Medina to the GCC citizens in hope of insulating itself from the pandemic (*Saudi Arabia temporarily suspends*, 2020).

When the first case was finally identified at the beginning of March, authorities introduced new restrictions: the Ministry of Sport suspended attendance at the sports events on the 6th of March (*Saudi Ministry of Sport suspends*, 2020), issued travel ban to European Union and 12 African and Asian countries (*Saudi Arabia expands*, 2020), introduced a lockdown, closing mosques and suspending public and private transportation on 20th of March (*Saudi Arabia bans*, 2020) and launching a periodic curfew in the entire realm on the 24th of March (Saudi Gazette 2020). WHO called to take immediate action to curb the spread of the novel coronavirus as numbers soar to 100 000 cases globally on the 7th of March, nevertheless it is not clear whether authorities of KSA acted in response to that call to action (*Critical preparedness*, 2020). It is unlikely, as the first major lockdown was introduced two days before WHO published guidelines for maintaining essential health services (*Operational guidance*, 2020). Nevertheless, the king's decree may be an effect of WHO's recommendations: on 30th of March King Salman issued a decree granting access to state-funded healthcare to all people currently living in the Kingdom, including the ex-pats and people who overstayed their visas (*Coronavirus: Saudi Arabia records*, 2020). It is worth noting that Saudi authorities were following WHO recommendations to curb the spread of fake news about the novel coronavirus (*Speech of the Director-General*, 2020), stating that attempts of spreading false information will be punished severely (*Coronavirus: Saudi Arabia reports*, 2020). On the 20th of March 18,7 billion USD, support package was announced to aid the private sector. On the 26th of March, the extraordinary G20 summit on COVID-19 took place, where global leaders were called to action to "find joint solutions and work together" (*WHO Director Generall calls*, 2020). The conference itself did not translate to immediate action on the Saudi part, nevertheless, some financial contributions were made at the end of the year.

April and May saw similar actions on the part of the government, mostly introducing periodic, local lockdowns (*Coronavirus: Saudi Arabia reimposes*, 2020) and curfews (Saudi Press Agency 2020; *Coronavirus: Saudi Arabia imposes*, 2020). Despite joint WHO and IMF April calls for lifting any restrictions in international trade of food and medicine, there was no immediate action on part of the Kingdom in that direction (*Press Release NO.20/187*, 2020). On the 15th of April G20 announced the adoption of a five-point Action Plan, one of which was launching the G20 Debt Service Suspension Initiative, a move highly praised by IMF Managing Director (*Press Release NO. 20/304*, 2020). Initially, 72 countries qualified for debt suspension. Originally it was to last only six months, nevertheless later this year it got extended.

Kingdom announced a three-phase re-opening plan on the 26th of May with actual re-opening happening in the middle of June (*Prophet Mosque to open*, 2020). During the holy month of Ramadan, restrictions were not lifted, as the authorities acted under WHO Safe Ramadan guidelines (*Safe Ramadan*, 2020). On the 10th of May government announced cuts in government employees' allowances to cover costs of living and tripled VAT from 5 to 15%, due to the fall in oil prices (*COVID-19 policy tracer, Saudi Arabia*, 2020).

June was also a month when the kingdom recorded the 100,000[th] case (*Coronavirus: Saudi Arabia now*, 2020). On the 21st of June major restrictions were lifted, with mosques being re-opened again and sports games restarted, without a live audience though (*Coronavirus: Mosques in Saudi Arabia's Mecca*, 2020). The same month WHO called for help from the international community to bring relief to the humanitarian crisis in Yemen (*Statement...*, WHO 2020). Saudi Arabia had taken steps that initially looked like the conflict that was ongoing since 2015 might come to an end (*As coronavirus spreads*, 2020): on the 9th of April the first ceasefire was announced, but it only lasted for two weeks (*Yemen War*, 2020). Fighting resumed in July (*Saudi-led coalition*, 2020). Saudi humanitarian conduct in Yemen announced before the 2020 G20 summit in Riyadh seems instrumental, nevertheless, it amounts to tangible help. July saw the launching of the G20 Debt Service Suspension Initiative, where G20 states (including KSA) decided to suspend debt repayments from 72 most vulnerable states, initiative was a part of the G20 Action plan announced on 15/04/2020 (*Press Release NO. 20/304*, 2020).

In July Saudi government opener land borders with GCC countries, 2nd of August 1000 pilgrims were allowed to perform the Hajj, and two days later commodity movement within GCC was re-started. By the end of August employees of the public sector, all came back to work (*COVID-19 policy tracer, Saudi Arabia*, 2020).

In September Saudi authorities were visibly trying to underline its global cooperation with other leaders in hopes of getting the vaccine, as King Salman had numerous conversations over the phone with Vladimir Putin, Angela Merkel, Francois Macron, Narendra Modi, and Xi Jin Ping. The same month's flights ban was also partially lifted, as the number of new cases started to decline significantly. As the G20 summit date was approaching Saudi Arabia announced its donation of 100 million USD to WHO (*Saudi Arabia backs*, 2020), and 46 million USD for 7 UNICEF projects in Yemen on behalf of King Salman Humanitarian Aid and Relief Centre (*Saudi Arabia KS Relief*, 2020). On the 29th of September, authorities announced allowing Umrah pilgrimage from the 4th of October (*Saudi Arabia to gradually resume*, 2020), under certain sanitary conditions.

5th of October was the first day on which the daily number of infections was lower than 400. The trend continued, and as a result on 10 of November authorities declared that the situation is stable, recommending wide-spread flu vaccination (*Saudi Arabia COVID-19 daily cases drop*, 2020) as a precautionary measure.

During the G20 Summit, held virtually in Riyadh, MBS underlined Saudi devotion to building a stronger and more sustainable world economy, at the same time pledging 500 million USD to fight COVID-19, it was Saudi share of 21 billion USD raised by G20 members (*Crown Prince*, 2020), consistently with IMF's call for solidarity with most vulnerable countries.

On the 17th of December, the COVID-19 vaccine campaign was launched in the kingdom (*Coronavirus: more than*, 2020). Within the first 24 hours government received over 300 000 applications (*Kingdom reports*, 2020). To promote the campaign on December 25th Crown Prince Mohammed ibn Salman received his vaccination live on national TV (*Saudi crown prince…*, 2020), two days later the number of vaccine registrations soared more than two-fold. By the end of December Ministry of Health announced that by February they plan to vaccine 1 million people (*Saudi Arabia to get 1m*, 2021).

Saudi Arabia seems to be one of the few countries in the Arab World which managed the pandemic exceptionally well comparing to the rest of the region. Despite the fact that it had the highest number of infections for a very long time, it maintained very high recovery rates, mainly to its well-funded healthcare system and adhering to the WHO and IMF recommendations. Saudi Arabia is a leader in the region in terms of the number of tests performed daily and is likely to remain stable politically and economically in foreseeable future. IMF predicted that the Saudi economy will start showing signs of recovery in the fourth quarter of 2020 (*COVID-19 policy tracer, Saudi Arabia*, 2020).

Case Study: Egypt

Egypt was the second state among the Arab League countries (after the United Arab Emirates) to have recorded a case of the coronavirus disease (Appendix 1), officially confirming it on the 14th of February. As recorded by WHO (*Egypt: WHO Coronavirus*, 2020), the state's biggest increase of new daily cases during the so-called first wave of the virus, fell on the period between the second half of May and the beginning of July with the highest number of new daily confirmed cases on June 20th reaching the number of 1,774 infections. After June 20th the numbers have reportedly started to decrease reaching a relatively steady pace of between a hundred and two hundred new cases a day. The situation began to escalate again in November, reaching another high in December with the highest record of the so-called second wave at 1,411 new cases noted on December 31st.

Figure 5. Daily New Cases in Egypt

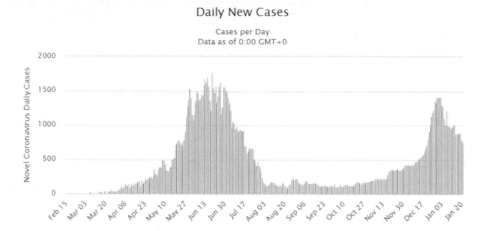

S o u r c e: Worldometer, https://www.worldometers.info/coronavirus/country/egypt, (Accessed: 22/01/2020.

When analyzing the state's response to SARS-COVID-2, it can be observed that Egypt falls into the group of 11 Arab League states (UAE, Tunisia, Oman, Mauretania, Morocco, Lebanon, Kuwait, Qatar, Jordan, Bahrain, Algeria) that did not decide on any preventive measures before the virus reached their borders (Attachment 3), despite many issued warnings and recommendations for preventive action and readiness (*Novel Coronavirus – Japan*, 2020) expressed by both WHO and IMF. The first case of infection in Egypt was recorded in mid-February, yet the first concrete measure imposed by the state in response to the virus occurred over a month later with the decision to close schools on March 15th (*Egypt: Country To Close Schools*, 2020) four days after WHO officially announced a global pandemic on March 11th. The time of the implementation of the prolonged response may have been coincidental, yet it was likely a direct effect of the situation being termed as a pandemic, which officially confirmed the danger and urgency of the situation at the same time making it more difficult for the government to stay silent and inactive due to a possible international and domestic pressure and accusation of negligence. However, before that, throughout February, the state did not remain completely silent but rather its response differed from what would be regarded as a common preventive measure imposed by states. In the early months of the discovery of the novel coronavirus, the global recommended action for countries evolved around supervising cases of influenza and respiratory infections, not restricting trade with China, sharing travel history (*Listings of WHO's responses*, 2020) with an additional focus on hand and respiratory hygiene, food safety, and avoidance of mass gatherings (*Mission summary*, 2020). In contrast, in the primary period of the pandemic, Egypt decided on a tactic of the containment of the spread of misinformation about the virus instead of the containment of the virus itself; as its first response (even before the closure of schools) it set up a hotline aimed at addressing misinformation (*Egypt's Health Ministry Receives*, 2020), a decision that does not find a clear correlation with the official global recommendations. WHO indeed did call for states to take action towards countering misinformation as early as February 3rd (*Listings of WHO's responses*, 2020), however, it seems unlikely that Egypt was acting in response to those recommendations, as they were primarily stressing the need to stop the spread of negative and false information about China as well as the conspiracies about the possible ways of transmission. Whereas in Egypt what the government perceived as misinformation was the broadcasted number of cases within the state, which the government claimed was smaller than advocated by the public. On March 1st, after already officially recording the first case of the disease, Prime Minister Mostafa Madbouly stated that there was "not a single coronavirus case on Egypt's soil" (*Saudi Arabia Closes Grand Mosque*, 2020). It may be inferred that instead of responding to WHO's postings and global recommendations, we can observe Egypt disregarding them by dismissing other calls like that of the call to not conceal the truth and to keep the population informed, aware, and actively involved in containment measures.

Other measures began to be imposed by Egypt in the second half of March and respectively included the suspension of international flights, partial closure of public places, and suspension of prayers. It may be observed that the time of the increase in measures after mid-March corresponded to the beginning of the second wave of infection within the country, therefore, may have been a response and an attempt of the government to limit the spread of cases. Similarly, the state activity increased - either new measures being imposed or their level of rigidity rising, for the duration of national and religious holidays as a temporary preventive measure. An example of which was witnessed during the Eid al-Adha holiday, for which Egypt increased its restrictions and for which similarly safe practice guidelines were also provided by WHO on July 25th (*Safe Eid al Adha*, 2020). However, WHO's recommendations remained to be rather general only suggesting that the cancellation of social and religious gatherings should be considered and that "any decision to restrict, modify, postpone, cancel, or proceed with holding a mass gathering should be based on a standardized risk assessment exercise, taking into account current epidemiological trends" (*Safe Eid al Adha*, 2020). Such a statement leaves a lot of room for the government's interpretation and it is therefore difficult to judge whether or not the preventive measures imposed in Egypt for the Eid al-Adha holiday were in any way guided and prompted by WHO's call.

In July the country went through a gradual lifting of restrictions, the main being the resumption of international flights after a three-month suspension and the reopening of the most strategic tourist attractions (*Egypt Reopens*, 2020). Respectively, every day throughout July Egypt noted a negative increase rate until August 6th. Therefore, a conclusion may be reached that the lifting of restrictions was a response to the internal circumstances of the country and respectively was also followed by a decline in new daily cases. There is no correlation found between Egypt's ease of restrictions and global recommendations as on July 31st WHO stated that "the Committee unanimously agreed that the pandemic still constitutes a public health emergency of international concern" (*Statement on the fourth meeting*, 2020) and called upon continuous engagement in combatting the virus. There have however also been calls for states to adhere to their internal circumstances, WHO underlined the responsibility of governments to "implement responses to the COVID-19 pandemic that are specific to their national context" (*Seventy Third World*, 2020). Therefore, there remains the question of the Egyptian government's adherence to national circumstances. The before mentioned correlation between easing the restrictions and the lower infection rate may be put to question as the infection rate ought to decrease earlier before the restrictions were already lifted for it to, could have truly been rooted in the situational context; a hypothesis that is supported by the issuing of the Government Reopening Plan, that was announced as early as in mid-May, in which the government was already beforehand planning the ease of restrictions that were to take place in June.

We are therefore driven to the conclusion that there is no clear and constant correlation between the responses of the state, be it the level of activity or the kind of measures being implemented, and the external recommendations coming from WHO or the IMF. The measures implemented by the government were more in line with the internal circumstances of the state than world events yet here it is necessary to stress that the apparent correlation may also be questionable due to Egypt's unconventional and self-contradicting tactics like that of running a disinformation campaign while supporting a conspiratorial discourse. Other unconventional measures included imprisonments for alleged misinformation, a 1% corona tax, and severe fines. It may therefore be speculated as to what extent the form of the government's response to internal circumstances was indeed prioritizing ending the spread of the virus over aiming at persevering and strengthening the ruling regime as well as its economic gains, especially in the tourism industry.

Conclusions

Based on the gathered data it can be stated that the virus was identified earliest in UAE and latest in Comoros, which does not mean that virus was brought in those places in that particular sequence. The most common places that virus was transmitted to the Arab World from are Iran, China, and Italy, which is hardly surprising due to the economic (China) and geographic (Iran and Italy) proximity of those countries. The highest overall number of infections was initially noted in KSA, Qatar, UAE, Kuwait, Egypt, Algeria, Bahrein, and Morocco. The number of identified infections seem to be growing along with the number of tests performed and because of that countries performing most test tend to have the highest number of cases as well. Just like in the other parts of the globe, the virus is most devastating for countries with low healthcare spendings and relatively high international air traffic (due to tourism or business). At first, the timing of taking preventive measures did not seem to matter, nevertheless with the current dynamic it looks like it may play a major role in combating the pandemic, for instance, KSA was one of the earliest responders, introducing restrictions way before the first case and seems to manage pandemic exceptionally well.

As of 31st of December 2021, Saudi Arabia is in third place in terms of the total number of cases, with Iraq being the first and Morocco the second, which again is highly correlated with the number of tests performed. The abrupt rise in the number of cases in the second half of 2020 across the region proves this point even further.

Data from most countries is incomplete at best, usually due to a lack of trustworthy information available in English. It should also be noted, that

Figure 6. The total number of cases on 31ˢᵗ of December 2020

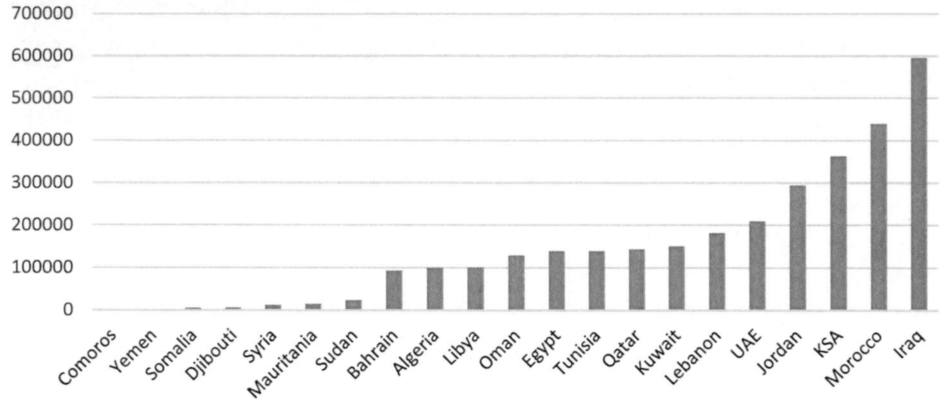

S o u r c e: based on https://www.worldometers.info/coronavirus/#countries.

the situation is the most worrying in countries where the number of cases is suspiciously low looking at the sizes of their populations, namely in Syria, Yemen, Sudan, and Somalia. Healthcare systems in those countries are on the verge of complete collapse, which in turn threatens overall well-being and in some cases even the survival of its populations in a long run.

International cooperation plays a crucial role in fighting the pandemic, as demonstrated with Gulf countries, governments of which adhered to the recommendations of WHO and contributed to the efforts aimed at providing relief by IMF. Saudi Arabia played a crucial role in that particular effort, being a host of two G20 summits that took place in 2020 and championing economic assistance to the countries in need. However, growing ambitions, as well as the more assertive approach to the regional security presented by the current Saudi government, contribute greatly to the economic and security hardship of the Yemeni population. Despite the danger that the pandemic poses to the entire Arab World, on-going conflicts there are far from being over. War in Yemen is a prime example of lack of ability to put the differences aside in the time of dire circumstances. That point is even more striking considering that GCC states managed to re-open their borders with Qatar at the same time. Much the same can be stated about the lack of decisive actions on the part of the Arab League, which is being continuously seen as an obscure and ineffective organization, that contributed very little to address the pandemic.

References

ACI World. (2015), *ACI World releases preliminary world airport traffic and rankings for 2014 – DXB becomes busiest airport for international passenger traffic* (2020), "Airports Council International", https://aci.aero/news/2015/03/26/aci-world-releases-preliminary-world-airport-traffic-and-rankings-for-2014-dxb-becomes-busiest-airport-for-international-passenger-traffic/,   (Accessed: 12.09.20).

IMF. (2020) *Policy Responses to COVID-19* (2020), https://www.imf.org/en/Topics/imf-and-covid19/Policy-Responses-to-COVID-19, (Accessed: 17/05/2021).

MacFarquahar N. (2011), *Arab League Votes to Suspend Syria Over Crackdown*, New York Times, 12/11/2011.

Our World in Data. (2020) *Number of Tests per country*, "Oxford University", https://ourworldindata.org/grapher/tests-of-covid-19-per-thousand-people-vs-gdp-per-capita?tab=table&year=latest&time=2020–09–09, (Accessed: 10/09/2020).

Tih F. (2020), *Comoros confirms 1st coronavirus case*, "AA", https://www.aa.com.tr/en/africa/comoros-confirms-1st-coronavirus-case/1825775,   (Accessed: 12/05/2020).

United Nations Development Programme, Human Development Report 2019 (2020), http://hdr.undp.org/sites/default/files/hdr2019.pdf,   (Accessed: 21/05/2020)., s. 308.

United Nations Development Programme, Human Development Report 2019 (2020), http://hdr.undp.org/sites/default/files/hdr2019.pdf,   (Accessed: 21/05/2020)., s. 308–311.

World Bank Population, total – Arab World, World (2020), https://data.worldbank.org/indicator/SP.POP.TOTL?locations=1A-1W, (Accessed: 20/05/2020).

World Bank, Current health expenditure per capita (current US$) - Saudi Arabia, United Arab Emirates, Qatar, Bahrain, Kuwait, Oman, Iraq, Egypt, Arab Rep., Lebanon (2020), https://data.worldbank.org/indicator/SH.XPD.CHEX.PC.CD?locations=SA-AE-QA-BH-KW-OM-IQ-EG-LB,   (Accessed: 22/05/2020).

World Bank, Current health expenditure per capita (current US$) - Syrian Arab Republic, Yemen, Rep., Mauritania, Comoros, Djibouti (2020), https://data.worldbank.org/indicator/SH.XPD.CHEX.PC.CD?locations=SY-YE-MR-KM-DJ, (Accessed: 21/05/2020).

World Bank, Current health expenditure per capita (current US$) - Arab World (2020), https://data.worldbank.org/indicator/SH.XPD.CHEX.PC.CD?locations=1A, (Accessed: 20/05/2020).

World Bank, Current health expenditure per capita (current US$) - Saudi Arabia, Qatar, Syrian Arab Republic, Comoros, Yemen, Rep., Iraq, Libya, Djibouti, So-

malia, Bahrain, Sudan, Mauritania, Jordan, Lebanon, Kuwait, Morocco, Tunisia, Oman, Egypt, Arab Rep., Algeria, United Arab Emirates (2020), https://data.worldbank.org/indicator/SH.XPD.CHEX.PC.CD?locations=SA-QA-SY-KM-YE-IQ-LY-DJ-SO-BH-SD-MR-JO-LB-KW-MA-TN-OM-EG-DZ-AE,   (Accessed: 17/05/2021).;

World Bank, GDP (current US$) – Arab World (2020), https://data.worldbank.org/indicator/NY.GDP.MKTP.CD?locations=1A, (Accessed: 20/05/2020).

World Bank, GDP (current US$) – European Union (2020), https://data.worldbank.org/indicator/NY.GDP.MKTP.CD?locations=EU, (Accessed: 20/05/2020).

World Bank, GDP (current US$) – India (2020), https://data.worldbank.org/indicator/NY.GDP.MKTP.CD?locations=1A-IN, (Accessed: 20/05/2020).

World Bank, GDP (current US$) – Saudi Arabia, Comoros (2020), https://data.worldbank.org/indicator/NY.GDP.MKTP.CD?locations=SA-KM,   (Accessed: 20/05/2020).

World Bank, GDP (current US$) - World (2020), https://data.worldbank.org/indicator/NY.GDP.MKTP.CD?locations=1A-1W, (Accessed: 20/05/2020).

World Bank, Mortality rate, infant (per 1,000 live births) - Saudi Arabia, Qatar, Syrian Arab Republic, Comoros, Yemen, Rep., Iraq, Libya, Djibouti, Somalia, Bahrain, Sudan, Mauritania, Jordan, Lebanon, Kuwait, Morocco, Tunisia, Oman, Egypt, Arab Rep., Algeria, United Arab Emirates (2020), https://data.worldbank.org/indicator/SP.DYN.IMRT.IN?locations=SA-QA-SY-KM-YE-IQ-LY-DJ-SO-BH-SD-MR-JO-LB-KW-MA-TN-OM-EG-DZ-AE, (Accessed: 17/05/2021).

Appendix 1
The sequence of identifying the first case in the Arab World.

Algerian health minister confirms first COVID-19 case (2020), "Africa Times", https://africatimes.com/2020)./02/25/algerian-health-minister-confirms-first-covid-19-case/, (Accessed: 12/05/2020).

Bahrain and Kuwait confirm first cases of coronavirus disease (2020), "Gulf News", https://gulfnews.com/world/gulf/bahrain/bahrain-and-kuwait-confirm-first-cases-of-coronavirus-disease-1.1582526120524, (Accessed: 12/05/2020).

Bahrain coronavirus case No. 1: A school bus driver (2020), "Gulf News", https://gulfnews.com/world/gulf/bahrain/bahrain-coronavirus-case-no-1-a-school-bus-driver-1.1582613552064, (Accessed: 12/05/2020).

Comoros confirms 1st coronavirus case (2020), "AA", https://www.aa.com.tr/en/africa/comoros-confirms-1st-coronavirus-case/1825775, (Accessed: 12/05/2020).

Coronavirus in UAE: Four of a family infected (2020), "Gulf News", https://gulfnews.com/uae/health/coronavirus-in-uae-four-of-a-family-infected-1.1580273983681, (Accessed: 12/05/2020).

Coronavirus Pandemic: A Timeline of COVID-19 in Morocco (2020), "Morocco World" News, https://www.moroccoworldnews.com/2020)./03/296727/corona-virus-a-timeline-of-covid-19-in-morocco/, (Accessed: 12/05/2020).

Coronavirus: Iraq, Oman confirm first cases, halt flights to Iran (2020), "The Strait Times", https://www.straitstimes.com/world/middle-east/coronavirus-iraq-con-firms-first-case, (Accessed: 12/05/2020).

Djibouti confirms first coronavirus case (2020), "The EastAfrican", https://www.theeastafrican.co.ke/scienceandhealth/Djibouti-confirms-first-coronavirus-case/3073694–5496666-ptn8nh/index.html, (Accessed: 12/05/2020).

Egypt announces first Coronavirus infection (2020), "Egypt Today", https://www.egypttoday.com/Article/01/81641/Egypt-announces-first-Coronavirus-infec-tion, (Accessed: 12/05/2020).

First Coronavirus Case Confirmed In Lebanon (2020), "The691", https://www.the961.com/first-coronavirus-in-lebanon/, (Accessed: 12/05/2020).

First Jordanian infected with coronavirus says he is recovering, cautions others (2020), "Al Arabiya", https://english.alarabiya.net/en/features/2020)./03/04/First-Jor-danian-infected-with-coronavirus-says-he-is-recovering-cautions-others.html, (Accessed: 12/05/2020).

Health Minister: First case of Coronavirus registered in Syria in patient who had come from abroad, appropriate measures have been taken to deal with the case (2020), "SANA", https://web.archive.org/web/2020).0322222624/https://sana.sy/en/?p=188671, (Accessed: 12/05/2020).

Italian returnee confirmed Tunisia's first coronavirus case (2020), "Punch", https://punchng.com/italian-returnee-confirmed-tunisias-first-coronavirus-case/, (Ac-cessed: 12/05/2020).

Libya confirms first coronavirus case amid fear over readiness (2020), "Reuters", https://www.reuters.com/article/us-health-coronavirus-libya-measures/libya-confirms-first-coronavirus-case-amid-fear-over-readiness-idUSKBN21B2SF, (Accessed: 12/05/2020).

Mauritania confirms first coronavirus case (2020), "CAN", https://www.channel-newsasia.com/news/world/mauritania-confirms-first-covid-19-coronavirus-case-12537688, (Accessed: 12/05/2020).

Novel Coronavirus (COVID-19): Iraq's Ministry of Health guidance to the public (2020), https://gds.gov.iq/novel-coronavirus-%e2%80%aacovid-19-iraqs-minis-try-of-health-guidance-to-the-public/, (Accessed: 12/05/2020).

Palestinians confirm first coronavirus cases in Gaza (2020), "AA", https://www.aa.com.tr/en/latest-on-coronavirus-outbreak/palestinians-confirm-first-coro-navirus-cases-in-gaza/1774636, (Accessed: 12/05/2020).

Qatar reports first case of coronavirus (2020), "The Peninsula", https://www.thepen-insulaqatar.com/article/29/02/2020)./Qatar-reports-first-case-of-coronavirus, (Accessed: 12/05/2020).

Saudi Arabia announces first case of coronavirus (2020), "Arab News", https://www.arabnews.com/node/1635781/saudi-arabia, (Accessed: 12/05/2020).

Somalia confirms first case of Covid-19 (2020), "The EastAfrican", https://www.theeastafrican.co.ke/scienceandhealth/Somalia-Covid-19-case/3073694–5493146-nx7h2b/index.html, (Accessed: 12/05/2020).

Sudan reports first coronavirus case (2020), "The EastAfrica", https://www.theeastafrican.co.ke/scienceandhealth/Sudan-reports-first-coronavirus-case/3073694–5489948-j7ya0lz/index.html, (Accessed: 12/05/2020).

Yemen 'faces nightmare' as first coronavirus case confirmed (2020), "BBC News", https://www.bbc.com/news/world-middle-east-52249624, (Accessed: 12/05/2020).

Appendix 2
Number of cases in each country as of 17th of May 2020

Coronavirus data for Algeria (2020), https://www.worldometers.info/coronavirus/country/algeria/, (Accessed: 17/05/2021).

Coronavirus data for Bahrein (2020), https://www.worldometers.info/coronavirus/country/bahrain/, (Accessed: 17/05/2021).

Coronavirus data for Comoros (2020), https://www.worldometers.info/coronavirus/country/comoros/, (Accessed: 17/05/2021).

Coronavirus data for Djibouti (2020), https://www.worldometers.info/coronavirus/country/djibouti/, (Accessed: 17/05/2021).

Coronavirus data for Egypt (2020), https://www.worldometers.info/coronavirus/country/egypt/, (Accessed: 17/05/2021).

Coronavirus data for Iraq (2020), https://www.worldometers.info/coronavirus/country/iraq/, (Accessed: 17/05/2021).

Coronavirus data for Jordan (2020), https://www.worldometers.info/coronavirus/country/jordan/, (Accessed: 17/05/2021).

Coronavirus data for Kuwait (2020), https://www.worldometers.info/coronavirus/country/kuwait/, (Accessed: 17/05/2021).

Coronavirus data for Lebanon (2020), https://www.worldometers.info/coronavirus/country/lebanon/, (Accessed: 17/05/2021).

Coronavirus data for Libya (2020), https://www.worldometers.info/coronavirus/country/libya/, (Accessed: 17/05/2021).

Coronavirus data for Mauritania (2020), https://www.worldometers.info/coronavirus/country/mauritania/, (Accessed: 17/05/2021).

Coronavirus data for Morocco (2020), https://www.worldometers.info/coronavirus/country/morocco/, (Accessed: 17/05/2021).

Coronavirus data for Oman (2020), https://www.worldometers.info/coronavirus/country/oman/, (Accessed: 17/05/2021).

Coronavirus data for Qatar (2020), https://www.worldometers.info/coronavirus/country/qatar/, (Accessed: 17/05/2021).

Coronavirus data for Saudi Arabia (2020), https://www.worldometers.info/coronavirus/country/saudi-arabia/, (Accessed: 17/05/2021).

Coronavirus data for Somalia (2020), https://www.worldometers.info/coronavirus/country/somalia/, (Accessed: 17/05/2021).

Coronavirus data for Sudan (2020), https://www.worldometers.info/coronavirus/country/sudan/, (Accessed: 17/05/2021).

Coronavirus data for Syria (2020), https://www.worldometers.info/coronavirus/country/syria/, (Accessed: 17/05/2021).

Coronavirus data for Tunisia (2020), https://www.worldometers.info/coronavirus/country/tunisia/, (Accessed: 17/05/2021).

Coronavirus data for UAE (2020), https://www.worldometers.info/coronavirus/country/united-arab-emirates/ (Accessed: 17/05/2020).

Coronavirus data for Yemen (2020), https://www.worldometers.info/coronavirus/country/yemen/, (Accessed: 17/05/2021).

Palestine confirms five more cases of COVID-19 (2020), "WAFA News Agency", https://english.wafa.ps/page.aspx?id=3QbJNWa117120820674a3QbJNW,   (Accessed: 17/05/2021).

Appendix 3
Type of restrictions introduced

Algeria: First COVID-19 fatality confirmed March 12/update 3 (2020), "Garda", https://www.garda.com/crisis24/news-alerts/322271/algeria-first-covid-19-fatality-confirmed-march-12-update-3, (Accessed: 17/05/2021).

Bahrain suspends all private, public schools amid coronavirus outbreak (2020), "Al Arabiya", http://english.alarabiya.net/en/News/gulf/2020)./02/25/Bahrain-suspends-all-private-public-schools-amid-coronavirus-outbreak.html, (Accessed: 17/05/2021).

Comoros: Authorities implement measure amid COVID-19 as of March 18 (2020), "GardaWorld", https://www.garda.com/crisis24/news-alerts/324541/comoros-authorities-implement-measures-amid-covid-19-as-of-march-18,   (Accessed: 17/05/2021).

Coronavirus pandemic: Experts say Somalia risk greater than China, "Al Jazeera", https://www.aljazeera.com/news/2020)./03/coronavirus-pandemic-experts-somalia-risk-greater-china-200319052938789.html, (Accessed: 17/05/2021).

COVID 19 Alert: Egypt closes Schools and Universities from March 15 (2020), "World Aware", https://www.worldaware.com/covid-19-alert-egypt-closes-schools-and-universities-march-15, (Accessed: 17/05/2021).

Dijbouti confirms first coronavirus case (2020), "The East African", https://www.theeastafrican.co.ke/scienceandhealth/Djibouti-confirms-first-coronavirus-case/3073694–5496666-ptn8nh/index.html, (Accessed: 17/05/2021).

Iraqi Government Imposes Curfew in Baghdad Over Coronavirus Concerns, (2020), "U.S. News", https://www.usnews.com/news/world/articles/2020).-03–15/iraqi-government-imposes-curfew-in-baghdad-over-coronavirus-concerns, (Accessed: 17/05/2021).

Jordan bars travelers from China, Iran, South Korea over virus (2020), "The Jakarta Post", https://www.thejakartapost.com/amp/travel/2020)./02/24/jordan-bars-travelers-from-china-iran-south-korea-over-virus.html, (Accessed: 17/05/2021).

Kuwait extends school closures for additional two weeks over coronavirus (2020), "Al Arabiya", https://english.alarabiya.net/News/gulf/2020/03/09/Coronavirus-Kuwait-extends-school-closures-for-additional-two-weeks-, (Accessed: 17/05/2021).

Lebanon asks schools and universities to close over coronavirus (2020), "Al Jazeera", https://www.aljazeera.com/news/2020)./02/lebanon-asks-schools-universities-close-coronavirus-200229152102382.html, (Accessed: 17/05/2021).

Libya announces raft of anti-corona virus measures (2020), "Libya Herald", https://www.libyaherald.com/2020)./03/17/libya-announces-raft-of-anti-corona-virus-measures/, (Accessed: 17/05/2021).

Mauritania: Authorities implement quarantine measures from travellers from China (2020), "GardaWorld", https://www.garda.com/crisis24/news-alerts/320091/mauritania-authorities-implement-quarantine-measures-for-travelers-from-china-as-of-february-5, (Accessed: 17/05/2021).

Morocco Suspends Schools Amid Coronavirus Fears (2020), "Morocco World News", https://www.moroccoworldnews.com/2020)./03/296119/morocco-suspends-school-amid-coronavirus-fears/, (Accessed: 17/05/2021).

Officials to close Syria-Kurdistan Region border to block coronavirus (2020), "Kurdistan24", https://www.kurdistan24.net/en/news/84714a1a-24c4–4854-bec3–09820b6f3cfb, (Accessed: 17/05/2021).

Passports Announces Suspension of Travel to China (2020), "Saudi Press Agency", https://www.spa.gov.sa/viewstory.php?lang=en&newsid=2031187, (Accessed: 17/05/2021).

Qatar suspends schools and universities due to coronavirus (2020), "The Pensinsula", https://www.thepeninsulaqatar.com/article/09/03/2020)./Qatar-suspends-schools-and-universities-due-to-coronavirus, (Accessed: 17/05/2021).

Sudan: Government closes borders due to COVID-19 on March 16 (2020), "GardaWorld", https://www.garda.com/crisis24/news-alerts/323581/sudan-government-closes-borders-due-to-covid-19-on-march-16-update-1, (Accessed: 17/05/2021).

Supreme Committee Takes More Decisions on Covid-19 Pandemic (2020), "Oman News Agency", https://omannews.gov.om/NewsDescription/ArtMID/392/ArticleID/10389/Supreme-Committee-Takes-More-Decisions-on-Covid-19-Pandemic, (Accessed: 17/05/2021).

Tunisia: Lockdown measures to ease from May 4 (2020), "GardaWorld", https://www.garda.com/crisis24/news-alerts/337711/tunisia-lockdown-measures-to-ease-from-may-4-update-8, (Accessed: 17/05/2021).

UAE schools to close from Sunday March 8 (2020), "TimeOutDubai", https://www.timeoutdubai.com/kids/435627-uae-schools-to-close-from-sunday-march-8, (Accessed: 17/05/2021).

Yemen: Saudi-backed government cancels flights for two weeks from March 18 over COVID-19 concerns (2020), "GardaWorld", https://www.garda.com/crisis24/news-alerts/322886/yemen-saudi-backed-government-cancels-flights-for-two-weeks-from-march-18-over-covid-19-concerns, (Accessed: 17/05/2021).

Appendix CIA FactBook

Data for Algeria (2020), „CIA", https://www.cia.gov/library/publications/the-world-factbook/geos/ag.html, (Accessed: 17/05/2021).

Data for Bahrain (2020), „CIA", https://www.cia.gov/library/publications/the-world-factbook/geos/ba.html, (Accessed: 17/05/2021).

Data for Comoros (2020), „CIA", https://www.cia.gov/library/publications/the-world-factbook/geos/cn.html, (Accessed: 17/05/2021).

Data for Djibouti (2020), „CIA", https://www.cia.gov/library/publications/the-world-factbook/geos/dj.html, (Accessed: 17/05/2021).

Data for Egypt (2020), „CIA", https://www.cia.gov/library/publications/the-world-factbook/geos/eg.html, (Accessed: 17/05/2021).

Data for Iraq (2020), „CIA", https://www.cia.gov/library/publications/the-world-factbook/geos/iz.html, (Accessed: 17/05/2021).

Data for Jordan (2020), „CIA", https://www.cia.gov/library/publications/the-world-factbook/geos/jo.html, (Accessed: 17/05/2021).

Data for Kuwait (2020), „CIA", https://www.cia.gov/library/publications/the-world-factbook/geos/ku.html, (Accessed: 17/05/2021).

Data for Lebanon (2020), „CIA", https://www.cia.gov/library/publications/the-world-factbook/geos/le.html, (Accessed: 17/05/2021).

Data for Libya (2020), „CIA", https://www.cia.gov/library/publications/the-world-factbook/geos/ly.html, (Accessed: 17/05/2021).

Data for Mauritania (2020), „CIA", https://www.cia.gov/library/publications/the-world-factbook/geos/mr.html, (Accessed: 17/05/2021).

Data for Morocco (2020), „CIA", https://www.cia.gov/library/publications/the-world-factbook/geos/mo.html, (Accessed: 17/05/2021).

Data for Oman (2020), „CIA", https://www.cia.gov/library/publications/the-world-factbook/geos/mu.html, (Accessed: 17/05/2021).

Data for Qatar (2020), „CIA", https://www.cia.gov/library/publications/the-world-factbook/geos/qa.html, (Accessed: 17/05/2021).

Data for Saudi Arabia (2020), „CIA", https://www.cia.gov/library/publications/the-world-factbook/geos/sa.html, (Accessed: 17/05/2021).

Data for Somalia (2020), „CIA", https://www.cia.gov/library/publications/the-world-factbook/geos/so.html, (Accessed: 17/05/2021).

Data for Sudan (2020), „CIA", https://www.cia.gov/library/publications/the-world-factbook/geos/su.html, (Accessed: 17/05/2021).

Data for Syria (2020), „CIA", https://www.cia.gov/library/publications/the-world-factbook/geos/sy.html, (Accessed: 17/05/2021).

Data for Tunisia (2020), „CIA", https://www.cia.gov/library/publications/the-world-factbook/geos/ts.html, (Accessed: 17/05/2021).

Data for UAE (2020), „CIA", https://www.cia.gov/library/publications/the-world-factbook/geos/ae.html, (Accessed: 17/05/2021).

Data for Yemen (2020), „CIA", https://www.cia.gov/library/publications/the-world-factbook/geos/ym.html, (Accessed: 17/05/2021).

Data on Saudi Arabia

As coronavirus spreads, U.N. seeks Yemen urgent peace talks resumption (2020), "Reuters", https://www.reuters.com/article/us-yemen-security/as-coronavirus-spreads-u-n-seeks-yemen-urgent-peace-talks-resumption-idUSKBN21K1P4, (Accessed: 14/10/2020).

Coronavirus: more than 700 000 register to receive vaccine in Saudi Arabia (2020), "Al Arabiya", https://english.alarabiya.net/en/coronavirus/2020)./12/27/Corona-virus-Coronavirus-More-than-700–000-register-to-receive-vaccine-in-Saudi-Arabia, (Accessed: 19/01/2020).

Coronavirus: Mosques in Saudi Arabia's Mecca set to reopen on June 21 (2020), "Al Arabiya", https://english.alarabiya.net/en/coronavirus/2020)./06/19/Coronavi-rus-Mosques-in-Saudi-Arabia-s-Mecca-set-to-reopen-on-June-21.html, (Accessed: 14/10/2020).

Coronavirus: Saudi Arabia imposes 24-hour curfew in several cities, including Riyadh (2020), "Al Arabiya", https://english.alarabiya.net/en/News/gulf/2020)./04/06/Coronavirus-Saudi-Arabia-imposes-24-hour-curfew-in-several-cities-includ-ing-Riyadh.html, (Accessed: 13/10/2020).

Coronavirus: Saudi Arabia now has over 100,000 COVID-19 cases (2020), "Al Arabiya", https://english.alarabiya.net/en/coronavirus/2020)./06/07/Coronavirus-Saudi-Arabia-now-has-more-than-100–000-COVID-19-cases-.html, (Accessed: 14/10/2020).

Coronavirus: Saudi Arabia records 1,453 cases (2020), "Al Arabiya", https://english.alarabiya.net/en/News/gulf/2020)./03/30/Coronavirus-Saudi-Arabia-records-1–453-cases.html, (Accessed: 12/10/2020).

Coronavirus: Saudi Arabia reimposes restrictions, curfew in Jeddah (2020), "Al Arabiya", https://english.alarabiya.net/en/coronavirus/2020)./06/05/Coronavirus-Saudi-Arabia-halts-all-workplace-attendance-in-Jeddah.html, (Accessed: 13/10/2020).

Coronavirus: Saudi Arabia reports first death, 205 new cases of COVID-19 (2020), "Gulf News", https://gulfnews.com/world/gulf/saudi/coronavirus-saudi-arabia-reports-first-death-205-new-cases-of-covid-19–1.1585054457152, (Accessed: 12/10/2020).

COVID-19 cases remain stable, flu vaccine recommended for all in Saudi Arabia (2020), "Arab News", https://www.arabnews.com/node/1760606/saudi-arabia, (Accessed: 06/01/2021).

Crown Prince Mohammad bin Salman: Saudi Arabia devoted G20 presidency to stronger, more sustainable world (2020), "Arab News", https://arab.news/45xq9, (Accessed: 06/01/2021).

G20 Debt Service Suspension Initiative, Press Release NO. 20/304, IMF News Library, https://www.imf.org/en/News/Articles/2020)./10/02/pr20304-imf-executive-board-extends-immediate-debt-service-relief-28-eligible-lics-six-months, (Accessed: 17/05/2021).

IMF COVID-19 policy tracer, Saudi Arabia (2020), https://www.imf.org/en/Topics/imf-and-covid19/Policy-Responses-to-COVID-19#S, (Accessed: 16/01/2021).

Kingdom reports 10 COVID-19 deaths as 300 000 register for vaccine (2020), "Arab News", https://www.arabnews.com/node/1779326/saudi-arabia, (Accessed: 19/01/2020).

Ministry of Interior: Curfew in All Makkah and Madinah for 24 Hours Effective from Today until Further Notice (2020), "Saudi Press Agency", https://www.spa.gov.sa/viewstory.php?lang=en&newsid=2054196, (Accessed: 13/10/2020).

Press Release NO. 20/304 (2020), "IMF News Library", https://www.imf.org/en/News/Articles/2020)./10/02/pr20304-imf-executive-board-extends-immediate-debt-service-relief-28-eligible-lics-six-months, (Accessed: 15/10/2020).

Prophet Mosque to open to public in stages from Sunday, "Arab News", https://www.arabnews.com/node/1681896/saudi-arabia, (Accessed: 13/10/2020).

Saudi Arabia backs UN's coronavirus response plan with 100 million USD (2020), "Arab News", https://www.arabnews.com/node/1736946/saudi-arabia, (Accessed: 05/01/2021).

Saudi Arabia bans prayers at mosques over coronavirus fears (2020), "Al Jazeera", https://www.aljazeera.com/news/2020)./3/20/saudi-arabia-bans-prayers-at-mosques-over-coronavirus-fears, (Accessed: 11/10/2020).

Saudi Arabia closes Grand Mosque, Prophet's Mosque between night and morning prayers (2020), "Arab News", https://www.arabnews.com/node/1637341/saudi-arabia, (Accessed: 10/10/2020).

Saudi Arabia COVID-19 daily cases drop below 400 for first time in six months (2020), "Arab News", https://www.arabnews.com/node/1744011/saudi-arabia, (Accessed: 05/01/2021.

Saudi Arabia COVID-19 testing (2020), "Our World in Data", https://ourworldindata.org/coronavirus/country/saudi-arabia?country=~SAU#are-countries-testing-enough-to-monitor-their-outbreak, (Accessed: 22/01/2020).

Saudi Arabia expands travel ban to and from EU, 12 more countries as coronavirus cases in Kingdom jump to 45 (2020), "Arab News", https://www.arabnews.com/node/1640286/saudi-arabia, (Accessed: 11/10/2020).

Saudi Arabia identifies first COVID-19 case (2020), "Arab News", https://www.arabnews.com/node/1635781/saudi-arabia, (Accessed: 10/10/2020).

Saudi Arabia KS Relief signs 46m USD deal with UNICEF for Yemen programs (2020), "Arab News", https://www.arabnews.com/node/1738091/saudi-arabia, Arab News, (Accessed: 05/01/2021).

Saudi Arabia Ministry of Health, COVID-19 (2020), https://covid19.moh.gov.sa/, (Accessed: 19/01/2020).

Saudi Arabia reports 51 new cases, total now 562 (2020), "Saudi Gazette", https://saudigazette.com.sa/article/591172/SAUDI-ARABIA/Saudi-Arabia-reports-51new-cases-total-now-562, (Accessed: 10/10/2020).

Saudi Arabia temporarily suspends entry of GCC citizens to Mecca and Medina: foreign ministry (2020), "Reuters", https://www.reuters.com/article/us-health-china-saudi-idUSKCN20M31T, (Accessed: 11/10/2020).

Saudi Arabia to get 1m Pfizer vaccines by February, records 11 COVID-19 deaths (2020), "Arab News", https://www.arabnews.com/node/1784011/saudi-arabia, (Accessed: 19/01/2020).

Saudi Arabia to gradually resume Umrah pilgrimage from October 4ᵗʰ (2020), "Arab News", https://www.arabnews.com/node/1738626/saudi-arabia, (Accessed: 05/01/2021).

Saudi Arabia will resume sports activities, without fans starting from June 21 (2020), "Reuters", https://www.reuters.com/article/us-health-coronavirus-saudi-sports/saudi-arabia-will-resume-sports-activities-without-fans-starting-from-june-21-idUSKBN23I3EQ, (Accessed: 14/10/2020).

Saudi crown prince receives first dose of Covid-19 vaccine (2020), "Middle Eastern Eye", https://www.middleeasteye.net/news/saudi-mbs-crown-prince-receives-first-dose-covid-19-vaccine, (Accessed: 19/01/2020).

Saudi Ministry of Sport suspends public attendance at events from Saturday (2020), "Arab News", https://www.arabnews.com/node/1637806/saudi-arabia, (Accessed: 11/10/2020).

Saudi-led coalition hits Houthi-held areas in renewed air raids (2020), "Al Jazeera", https://www.aljazeera.com/news/2020)./7/2/saudi-led-coalition-hits-houthi-held-areas-in-renewed-air-raids, (Accessed: 15/10/2020).

Speach of the Director General at Munich Security Conference (2020), "WHO", https://www.who.int/director-general/speeches/detail/munich-security-conference, (Accessed: 12/10/2020).

Statement from Dr Mike Ryan, Executive Director, WHO Health Emergencies Programme at the Yemen High-level Pledging Conference. 2 June (2020), "WHO", https://www.who.int/news/item/02–06–2020-statement-from-dr-mike-ryan-executive-director-who-health-emergencies-programme-at-the-yemen-high-level-pledging-conference 2020, (Accessed: 14/10/2020).

Safe Ramadan practices in the context of the COVID-19: interim guidance (2021), "WHO", https://www.who.int/publications/i/item/safe-ramadan-practices-in-the-context-of-the-covid-19-interim-guidance, (Accessed: 19/01/2020).

WHO and IMF call for lifting restrictions on trading food and medicine, Press Release NO.20/187, (2020) "IMF News Library", https://www.imf.org/en/News/Articles/2020)./04/24/pr20187-wto-and-imf-joint-statement-on-trade-and-the-covid-19-response, (Accessed: 17/05/2021).

WHO Director-General calls on G20 to Fight, Unite, and Ignite against COVID-19 (2020) "WHO",, https://www.who.int/news/item/26–03–2020-who-s-director-general-calls-on-g20-to-fight-unite-and-ignite-against-covid-19,   (Accessed: 12/10/2020).

WHO.COVID-19: Operational guidance for maintaining essential health services during an outbreak (2020), Interim guidance 25 March 2020, (2020), "WHO",https://www.who.int/publications/i/item/strategic-planning-and____operational-guidance-for-maintaining-essential-health-services-during-an-outbreak (Accessed: 12/10/2020).

Critical preparedness, readiness and response actions for COVID-19: interim guidance (2021), "WHO", https://apps.who.int/iris/handle/10665/331422, (Accessed: 11/10/2020).

COVID-19 in Saudi Arabia (2020), Worldometer, https://www.worldometers.info/coronavirus/country/saudi-arabia/, (Accessed: 19/01/2020).

Yemen war: Coalition ceasefire to help combat coronavirus begins (2020), https://www.bbc.com/news/world-middle-east-52224358, (Accessed: 14/10/2020).

Data on Egypt

Saudi Arabia Closes Grand Mosque, Prophet'S Mosque Between Night And Morning Prayers (2021), "Arab News", https://www.arabnews.com/node/1637341/saudi-arabia, (Accessed: 5/01/2021).

Egypt: WHO Coronavirus Disease (COVID-19) Dashboard (2021), "WHO", https://covid19.who.int/region/emro/country/eg, (Accessed: 5/01/2021).

Egypt's Health Ministry Receives Over 344K Calls Via COVID-19 Hotlines In March (2021), "Egypt Today", https://www.egypttoday.com/Article/01/83384/Egypt-s-Health-Ministry-receives-over-344k-calls-via-COVID, (Accessed: 1/01/2021).

Egypt Faces Stricter Lockdown Measures For The Week Of Eid El Fitr Before Phase 1 Of Gov'T Reopening Plan Comes Into Effect (2021), "Enterprise", https://enterprise.press/stories/2020)./05/18/egypt-faces-stricter-lockdown-measures-for-the-week-of-eid-el-fitr-before-phase-1-of-govt-reopening-plan-comes-into-effect-16083/, (Accessed: 1/01/2021).

Egypt: Country To Close Schools, Universities For Two Weeks From March 15 Over COVID-19 Concerns /Update 6 (2021*)*, "GardaWorld", https://www.garda.com/crisis24/news-alerts/322876/egypt-country-to-close-schools-universities-for-two-weeks-from-march-15-over-covid-19-concerns-update-6, (Accessed: 5/01/2021).

Egypt Reopens Airports And Welcomes Tourists To Pyramids After COVID Closure (2020), "U.S. News", https://www.usnews.com/news/world/articles/2020).-07–01/egypt-reopens-airports-and-welcomes-tourists-to-pyramids-after-covid-closure, (Accessed: 3/11/2021).

Listings of WHO's response to COVID-19. Statement. Last updated 15 December 2020. (2020), "WHO", https://www.who.int/news/item/29–06–2020-covidtimeline, (Accessed: 17/05/2021).

Listings of WHO's response to COVID-19. Statement. Last updated 15 December 2020 (2020), "WHO", https://www.who.int/news/item/29–06–2020-covidtimeline, (Accessed: 17/05/2021).

Mission summary: WHO Field Visit to Wuhan (2020), China 20–21 January 2020, "WHO".

Seventy-Third World Health Assembly: Covid-19 Response. Agenda item 3, 19 May 2020, (2020), "WHO", https://apps.who.int/gb/ebwha/pdf_files/WHA73/A73_R1-en.pdf, (Accessed: 3/01/2021).

Statement on the fourth meeting of the International Health Regulations (2005) Emergency Committee regarding the outbreak of coronavirus disease (COVID-19), (2020), "WHO", https://www.who.int/news/item/01–08–2020-statement-on-the-fourth-meeting-of-the-international-health-regulations-(2005)-emergency-committee-regarding-the-outbreak-of-coronavirus-disease-(covid-19), (Accessed: 17/05/2021).

Listings Of WHO's Response To COVID-19 (2021), "WHO", https://www.who.int/news/item/29–06–2020-covidtimeline, (Accessed: 5/01.2021).

WHO Director-General's Opening Remarks At The Media Briefing On COVID-19 - 11 March 2020, (2021), "WHO", https://www.who.int/director-general/speeches/detail/who-director-general-s-opening-remarks-at-the-media-briefing-on-covid-19---11-march-2020, (Accessed: 7/01/2021).

Safe Eid al Adha practices in the context of COVID-19: interim guidance (2020), "WHO", World Health Organization. https://apps.who.int/iris/handle/10665/333454. License: CC BY-NC-SA 3.0 IGO, (Accessed: 17/05/2021).

Novel Coronavirus – Japan (Ex-China) (2021), "WHO", https://www.who.int/csr/don/16-january-2020-novel-coronavirus-japan-ex-china/en/, (Accessed: 7/01/2021).

Przemysław Osiewicz
Adam Mickiewicz University, Poznań
https://orcid.org/0000-0001-6883-7307

THE COVID-19 PANDEMIC IN IRAN: MANAGING PANDEMIC THREAT UNDER POLITICAL AND ECONOMIC SANCTIONS[1]

Introduction

The appearance of the COVID-19 virus came as a surprise to the international community, even though it was not the first and certainly not the last time such a virus appeared. Initially, no country in the world was prepared to limit its spread and the number of infected patients. It was not clear how is the virus transmitted, what is the incubation time, on which materials it can survive shorter and longer. Thus, it was not clear for a long time what measures should be implemented in order to deal effectively with the new threat. This concerned both material measures and measures to limit social contacts. The World Health Organization (WHO) has amended its recommendations to member states several times. The Islamic Republic of Iran necessarily was in the same situation as it tried to adjust its health care system and the activities of other state services to the current WHO guidelines.

The purpose of this chapter is to analyze the course of the epidemic and the measures introduced by the Iranian authorities to limit it under the conditions of political and economic sanctions imposed on the country. The main research questions are as follows:

- What social measures were applied to counteract the epidemic threat?

---

[1] The research was financed from the project „Research on COVID-19" from the funds of the Adam Mickiewicz University, Poznan

- What economic measures were applied to counteract the epidemic threat?
- Were the introduced restrictions and recommendations consistent with the recommendations of the World Health Organization?
- Have the political and economic sanctions imposed on Iran impeded the fight against the epidemic threat? If yes, to what extent?

The main research technique is qualitative content analysis. The types of political and economic measures applied to counteract the epidemic threat are the main research tool. As for the structure and division of the chapter content, the first part is dedicated to a detailed analysis of the course of the pandemic in Iran. Social and economic measures applied to counteract the epidemic threat in Iran are presented in the second part. The last part attempts to identify the relationship between the restrictions introduced and the methods of counteracting the spread of the epidemic in Iran and the sanctions, especially economic ones, imposed on this country.

The course of the pandemic in Iran

The first confirmed cases of COVID-19 infections in Iran were reported on 19 February 2020 (Abdi, 2020: 1) in the city of Qom, which is an important center of religious education and a place of pilgrimage. In the days that followed the virus spread rapidly both in and around Qom Province, especially in the capital city of Tehran.

The pace at which the virus spread to Iran was significantly influenced by missed or too late decisions. In the early stages of the epidemic, a significant mistake was made with the announcement of a few days off to prevent the spread of the pandemic. Many Iranians used their days off as usual and massively went on trips or vacation stays. An additional factor was a very bad information policy, especially the comparison of the COVID-19 virus with the common flu virus, which was spread in the public media (Arab-Zozani, Ghoddoosi-Nejad, 2020: 2). All these factors, which occurred at the same time, translated into an exceptionally rapid increase in the number of cases and a serious crisis in the Iranian health care system. At that time, there were no clear indications for all possible routes of transmission of the infection and the most effective methods of preventing infection. WHO has modified its positions several times.

As of 8 March 2021, there were 1,689,692 reported cases of COVID-19 infection in Iran, 1,442,198 people recovered and 60,687 people died. The mortality rate in the group of so-called closed cases was 4 percent (*Iran coronavirus*, 2021). After nearly a year, the pandemic situation has become stable. Nevertheless, for the first few months of the threat, Iran was among the world's leading countries with the highest rates of morbidity and mortality. What factors led to this situation?

Measures applied to counteract the epidemic threat

The scale of the threat and the speed with which the virus spread in Iran and other countries in the region forced the executive authorities to take swift institutional and organizational measures. At the institutional level, the most important activity was the creation of the National Committee on Combating Coronavirus. According to the official information provided to the U.S. National Library of Medicine by the Iranian Ministry of Health and Medical Education, "this Committee is official source of gathering, analyzing, and reporting the COVID-19 data in Iran. The data of all sources in the country including, medical care monitoring center (MCMC), Hospitals' Information Systems (HIS), Laboratory portal, the data of the center for communicable disease control (MOH), as well as the data from community health centers are integrated and used in this regards" (*Daily situation report*, 2020).

Shortly after the sudden increase in the number of cases in early March 2020, the Iranian Ministry of Health and Medical Education applied the following measures to stop the spread of the virus:
- raising public awareness of the epidemic threat and recommendations proposed by the World Health Organization to stop COVID-19 infection, including: promoting frequent hand washing and the use of alcohol-containing virucides, keeping a minimum distance of one meter in relation to people who cough or have a cold, avoiding touching faces, eyes and mouth with contaminated hands, obligatory covering of mouth and nose by sick people in public places and seeking medical help in case of breathing problems, high fever or persistent cough;
- limiting the movement and flow of people in places with particularly high traffic, such as pilgrimage centers, tourist attractions and bazaars
- closing of kindergartens, schools and universities;

- limiting the number of working hours;
- cancellation of the congregational prayer and Jumu'ah prayer, namely the Friday prayer;
- cancellation of all team sport matches like football and volleyball;
- regular disinfection of public utility places and means of public transport;
- introduction of entry restrictions to detect people who may be infected at the entrances and exits of a number of cities;
- creation of groups and teams to diagnose the disease through district health centers located in different areas of the affected cities (Abdi, 2020: 1).

Although most of the aforementioned measures to counter the spread of the COVID-19 virus were in line with WHO recommendations and the practice of many countries, their implementation in Iran faced a number of obstacles, mainly of an organizational and financial nature. Among the main problems faced by the Iranian administration were: lack of specialized medical equipment and modern hospital infrastructure with a sufficient number of beds, difficulties importing essential equipment and medicines, unsuccessful attempts to quarantine individual cities due to the already very large number of cases recorded throughout the country, and increased risk of virus transmission caused by increased travel due to the New Year holiday – Nowruz – around 19 March 2020 (Abdi, 2020: 1–2).

The problems in fighting the epidemic were not only financial shortages and poor organization of the public health service. In the opinion of Morteza Arab-Zozani and Djavad Ghoddoosi-Nejad, "concurrent with questionable actions of the public authorities, some opportunistic jobbers who claimed traditional medicine, they called it Islamic medicine, prescribed various alternative solutions that were in contrast with the practice of modern scientific medicine. This, alongside a bewilderment of public authorities, resulted in a confused population, which added to the ill handling of controlling the pandemic" (Arab-Zozani, Ghoddoosi-Nejad, 2020: 2). Thus, the Iranian society has convinced itself of the importance of access to proven and credible expert knowledge. The lack of proper information by the executive authorities has led to misunderstandings and misinterpretation of the recommendations. The trust of some citizens in traditional medicine also played a negative role.

As in many other developing countries, one of the greatest social challenges has been to ensure universal access to education in the new context of compulsory distance learning. All schools and universities were already closed in the first phase of the pandemic in early March. This decision was fully justified and was in line with similar decisions in other countries affected by a sudden spike in the number of cases. In practice, however, it was associated with the actual deprivation of access to education for many children and students, especially in smaller urban centers and in the countryside. In poverty areas, there is not only a lack of access to computer equipment and the Internet, but even to television. The situation worsened further with the compulsory use of the official SHAD education platform for all teachers and students in Iran. The use of foreign applications such as Telegram and WhatsApp, commonly used by Iranian teachers until that time, was prohibited. Perhaps it would not be anything special, especially taking into account the specific approach of the Iranian authorities to the issue of security, were it not for the fact that the SHAD application only worked properly on phones with the latest version of Android installed. In addition, many users reported problems logging in to the website, numerous errors and a very slow data transfer. In the opinion of Alijani Ershad, "poverty is the principal problem for distance learning in the country. According to Iran's parliamentary research centre, between 40 and 55% of Iranians live under the poverty line. About 80% of Iranian internet users live in cities and around 20% in rural areas (Ershad, 2020).

After a few months, the negative effects of the first wave were brought under control. As in many European and Middle Eastern countries, the Iranian authorities began lifting the restrictions introduced in March. Such actions turned out to be premature and wrong. According to Amir Abdoli, "removing the restrictions in early May 2020 led to the beginning second wave of the disease with an increase number of cases in early June 2020 and a surge in the number of deaths on 15 June 2020. According to the last reports from the WHO, the third wave of the disease in Iran began in the early September 2020" (Abdoli, 2020). Thus, the third wave of the pandemic occurred faster in Iran than in Europe. This time the Iranian authorities were better prepared for the threat, but the shortages of medical equipment and personal protective equipment were still very noticeable.

Some analysts have pointed to a link between Iran's inadequate response to the first and second waves of the pandemic and the extended political and economic sanctions imposed on Iran by the United States after the Americans withdrew from the nuclear deal in 2018. Others have argued that the organization of public health services and the situation in Iran is bad even without considering the possible impact of the sanctions. Elham Ahmadn-ezdah and members of his research team were among them. In their opinion, "even before COVID-19, Iran's health system was feeling the effect of the sanctions. Their impact is now severe because they restrict the government's ability to raise funds or to import essential goods. Of the ten countries with the highest number of recorded cases of COVID-19 to date, Iran is the poorest" (Ahmadnezdah et al., 2020). Is it really possible to see a correlation between the sanctions in force and the course of the pandemic in Iran? Or maybe other researchers and analysts are right in their opinion that the sanctions are treated by the Iranian authorities as an instrumental explanation of their own wrong decisions?

Have the political and economic sanctions imposed on Iran impeded the fight against the epidemic threat?

Iran's political position in the international arena is different from that of many other developing countries. In terms of social development and stable economic growth, the biggest problem is connected with the extended sanctions imposed on Iran by the United States in 2018, after the U.S. administration withdrew from the Joint Comprehensive Plan of Action (JCPOA). In practice, these sanctions apply to all economic entities cooperating with Iranian partners under the threat of cutting off access to the American market. Any European or Asian concern, while continuing to cooperate with the Iranians, must take into account serious problems and restrictions from the United States. Serious restrictions in the sale of crude oil and natural gas, as well as a reduction in the inflow of foreign investments, significantly reduced budget revenues. Consequently, the possibilities for financing public health care have decreased, which has become particularly visible during the ongoing pandemic. However, opinions on this issue are divided. Some point to the negative impact of the sanctions, while others see the sources of high mortality and inefficiency in the Iranian health service in mismanagement and communication chaos. So which side is right? What arguments are being invoked in support of the thesis that the sanctions have a significant impact on the efficiency of the Iranian health service, and what are the opinions about its bad organization?

Some analysts on the Iranian political scene have harshly criticized the actions taken by the Iranian executive to counter the spread of the virus in the first weeks of the pandemic in February and March 2020. While pointing to the negative impact of economic sanctions on the effectiveness of the measures taken, they also emphasized that they were not the main cause of failure and the high number of fatalities in that period. In the opinion of Anicée Van Engeland, "Iran's lack of a coordinated response to the COVID-19 crisis combined with a slow decision-making process has had terrible consequences on society. While US sanctions are certainly an issue in terms of access to medical materials and medicine, the way the authorities have tackled the crisis raises questions. Preparing the country, including its medics, for a possible military conflict, including preparations for ground and air attacks across society, has consumed efforts" (Van Engeland, 2020).

On the other hand, there are scholars and analysts who disagree and see the significant impact of the political and economic sanctions on the effectiveness of the actions taken by the Iranian authorities to combat the epidemic threat and provide medical assistance to infected citizens. One of them is Amir Abdoli. In his opinion, "providing health services is one of the problems of Iran's health system during the COVID-19 crisis. The US sanctions against Iran compromised Iran's health system. Although the short time effects of sanctions may be negligible, the chronic and long-term effects of sanctions may be more tangible than their acute impact. Hence, beyond the harsh effects of political and economic sanctions against Iran, the country's health system is more jeopardized and need to be free from sanctions for battling against this crisis" (Abdoli, 2020: 4). Djavad Salehi-Isfahani is of a similar opinion. According to him, the pandemic "caught Iran at its weakest economic state since the end of the war with Iraq three decades ago. Since U.S.'s withdrawal from JCPOA in 2018, Iran's GDP has declined by 11 percent and average living standards (measured by real household per capita expenditure) have declined by 13 percent" (Salehi-Isfahani, 2020).

It is worth noting, however, that not all members of the Western world have left the Iranian authorities without aid. Despite the applicable US sanctions and restrictions, the European Union offered immediate aid to Iran. On 11 April 2020, Josep Borrell announced a new Team Europe project, aimed at helping the EU's partner countries in their fight against the effects of the COVID-19 pandemic. The amount initially declared was EUR 20 billion (Borrell, 2020). According to a fact sheet from the EU, 12.3 billion euro will be spent on mitigating the economic and social impact, 2.8 billion euro will go toward strengthening research and health systems, and 502 million euro will be dedicated to the short-term emergency response, to be directed to vulnerable communities in Africa, the Middle East, parts of Asia, Latin America, the Caribbean, and elsewhere (*EU global response*, 2020). The European External Action Service declared on its website: "The coronavirus has not only Europe but the entire global community in its grip and is the world's common enemy. An enemy we can only defeat with a global approach and cross-border coordination. And while we have to mobilize all our resources to fight the virus at home, now is also the time to look beyond our borders" (Team Europe, 2020). Among the beneficiaries in the MENA region, Jordan and Lebanon are to receive 240 million euro to support their citizens and Syrian refugees. Iran will get 20 million euro in emergency support. Refugees in Turkey will be provided with small-scale health infrastructure and equipment worth 90 million euro.

Conclusion

In 2020, Iran was one of the countries most affected by the COVID-19 pandemic, especially in terms of the number of cases and deaths. Counteracting the spread of the virus throughout the country overlapped with Iran's previous serious problems, both political and economic. In this case international politics has a significant influence on the resources and possibilities at the disposal of the Iranian authorities.

The political and economic sanctions imposed on Iran, especially in the period after the withdrawal of the United States from the nuclear deal with Iran in 2018, significantly impeded counteracting the epidemic threat in that country. As a consequence of the introduction of the so-called extended sanctions by the American administration, the possibility of sending the necessary drugs, medical equipment and medical supplies to the country was limited. Iran received aid from the European Union, but it was well below real needs.

Yet sanctions cannot be identified as the main cause of the failure and difficulties of the Iranian authorities in fighting the pandemic, especially during the first wave of the epidemic in spring 2020. The pandemic has demonstrated the need for urgent systemic reform of the Iranian health service and information policy of public administration bodies.

There is no doubt, however, that the sanctions have made it difficult for Iran to deal with the epidemic threat. To best prepare for possible future COVID-19 virus outbreaks or similar threats in the future, both sides should be prepared to make some concessions on issues that may affect first aid and life-saving opportunities. The international community, with particular emphasis on the United States, should modify the sanctions system in such a way that it will not hinder the transfer or sale of medical equipment, personal protective equipment and medicines to Iranian entities. Iranian authorities should be more open to the possibility of using experience, hardware and software (remote education) developed by companies from Western countries.

References

Abdi M. (2020), *Coronavirus disease 2019 (COVID-19) outbreak in Iran: Actions and problems*, "Infection Control and Hospital Epidemiology", Vol. 41, No. 6.

Abdoli A. (2020), *Iran, sanctions, and the COVID-19 crisis*, "Journal of Medical Economics", Vol. 24, No. 1.

Ahmadnezdah E., Murphy A., Abdi Z., Harirchi I., McKee M. (2020), *Economic sanctions and Iran's capacity to respond to COVID-19*, "The Lancet", Vol. 5, No. 5.

Arab-Zozani M., Ghodoosi-Nejad D. (2020), *COVID-19 in Iran: the Good, the Bad, and the Ugly Strategies for Preparedness – A Report From the Field*, "Disaster Medicine and Public Health Preparedness" Jul 27: 1–3.

Borrell J. (2020), https://twitter.com/JosepBorrellF/status/1248917498638020618 (Accessed:: 17.02.2021).

Daily Situation Report on Coronavirus disease (COVID-19) in Iran (2020), Archives of Academic Emergency Medicine, 25.03.2020, https://www.ncbi.nlm.nih.gov/pmc/articles/PMC7114715/ (Accessed:: 10.02.2021).

Ershad A. (2020), *In Iran, poverty and lack of internet make distance learning impossible*, France24, 21.04.2020, https://observers.france24.com/en/20200421-iran-internet-covid19-distance-learning-poverty (Accessed:: 12.02.2021).

EU global response to coronavirus: supporting our partner countries (2020), European Commission, 8.04.2020, https://ec.europa.eu/commission/presscorner/detail/en/fs_20_607 (Accessed:: 17.02.2021).

Iran coronavirus (2021), Worldometers, 8.03.2021, https://www.worldometers.info/coronavirus/country/iran/ (Accessed:: 8.03.2021).

Salehi-Isfahani J. (2020), *Iran: The double jeopardy of sanctions and COVID-19*, Brookings, 23.09.2020, https://www.brookings.edu/opinions/iran-the-double-jeopardy-of-sanctions-and-covid-19/ (Accessed:: 17.02.2021).

"Team Europe" - Global EU Response to Covid-19 supporting partner countries and fragile populations (2020), The European External Action Service, 11.04.2020, https://eeas.europa.eu/headquarters/headquarters-homepage/77470/%E2%80%9Cteam-europe%E2%80%9D-global-eu-response-covid-19-supporting-partner-countries-and-fragile-populations_en (Accessed:: 18.02.2021).

Van Engeland A. (2020), *Iran and COVID-19*, Cranfield University, 2.04.2020, https://www.cranfield.ac.uk/press/news-2020/iran-and-covid-19 (Accessed:: 12.02.2021).

Jarosław Kardaś
Adam Mickiewicz University, Poznan
0000-0002-1517-6215

FIGHTING THE COVID-19 PANDEMIC IN THE FORMER USSR AREA (A CASE OF THE COUNTRIES OF THE EURASIAN ECONOMIC UNION)[1]

Introduction

The COVID-19 pandemic has hit the post-Soviet countries very hard (Legieć, 2020a). In the Russian Federation alone, more people lost their lives by the end of 2020 as a result of the pandemic than during the 1939–1940 war with Finland. It is worth noting, however, that the real number of coronavirus victims in the region may be much higher, as falsification of relevant statistics has been (and still is) commonplace in Russia and other post-Soviet republics. A notable case in point is Bashkiria (located in the southern part of Russia), a country of 4 million people, where only 70 people have officially died (by the beginning of December) from coronavirus (Radziwinowicz, 2020). The largely ineffective fight against COVID-19 in the post-Soviet region is not only a result of internal problems of the countries situated in the area (such as underfunded health services) but also the weakness of integration structures, which do not make the fight against this biological threat any easier. Two research hypotheses were developed for this article. The first one assumes that cooperation of the countries forming the Eurasian Economic Union in tackling the COVID-19 pandemic has been ineffective because the

---

[1] The research was financed from the project „Research on COVID-19" from the funds of the Adam Mickiewicz University, Poznan

Russian Federation (as the country with the strongest position within this structure) has helped the other members only within the framework of bilateral relations, rather than through the structures of this organization. This assistance resulted from vested Russian interests rather than solidarity considerations towards the post-Soviet states. The other hypothesis states that the low effectiveness of the Eurasian Economic Union's efforts to combat the pandemic has led to individual member states having to develop ways to fight coronavirus at their own (national) levels. The article applies the institutional-legal method and the fact-finding method. They were used to describe the actions taken within the Eurasian Economic Union and also to characterize the restrictions introduced by the authorities of Armenia, Belarus, Kazakhstan, Kyrgyzstan, and Russia during the pandemic.

The Eurasian Economic Union's response to the COVID-19 pandemic

The Eurasian Economic Union (EEU) is an integration project for the post-Soviet area that was initiated by the Russian Federation. One of the first decisions in the fight against coronavirus was taken by the Eurasian Economic Union on 16 March 2020. It was decided that customs duties would be abolished on goods imported in order to prevent the spread of coronavirus in the EEU countries. This has primarily concerned personal protective equipment, disinfectants, as well as certain types of medical equipment and medical materials. Then, on 24 March, a temporary ban was imposed on the export of personal protective equipment, disinfectants, medical products, and other materials needed to fight coronavirus from the Eurasian Economic Union countries. This included masks, respirators, filters used for respiratory protection, goggles, bandages, disinfectants, and gloves. On 25 March, in turn, the member states committed to exchange information and consult on internal legislation to fight coronavirus. In addition, the Eurasian Economic Union members were to coordinate the activities of bodies with competence in health protection and those responsible for the sanitary-epidemiological sphere. It was also decided that in case one of the member states was short of medical equipment to fight the pandemic, the other members would arrange adequate shipments to that country (Обзор, 2020). On 10 April 2021, the Eurasian Intergovernmental Council adopted an order on community action to stabilize the economic situation in the member states. An assistance program developed by the Commission was designed to minimize the consequences for business, sustain employment in the most sensitive industries, and ensure the stability of financial systems in the member states (Обзор, 2020).

The ban on the export of certain types of personal protective equipment, protective and disinfectant products, medical products, and materials from the countries of the Eurasian Economic Union, which was introduced in the spring of 2020, ceased to apply from 1 October 2020. Another important decision within the Eurasian Economic Union was also taken on 1 October. It was decided that the duty-free import regime on the EEU territory for individual components and materials needed for the production of medicines and disinfectants, as well as respirators, protective goggles, rubber gloves, and other types of medical equipment, will be extended until 31 March 2021 (Обзор, 2020).

Looking at the actions of the Eurasian Economic Union in the face of the COVID-19 pandemic, it can be concluded that they are ineffective and do not contribute to the development of cooperation between its members. This is partly due to the fact that for several years Russia itself has been primarily concerned about political integration rather than tightening economic relations, which other members of the organization have been seeking (Legieć, 2020a). This can be seen, for example, in the actions taken after the decision to ban exports of medical equipment, protective clothing, and cleaning and disinfecting products to other countries. The decision was not respected by the Russian Federation, as demonstrated by the situation that occurred at the beginning of the pandemic in Kyrgyzstan. There was a considerable shortage of medical supplies in the republic, which unfortunately resulted in the deaths of much medical personnel. The country's authorities made an official request to the Russian Federation to support Kyrgyzstan and send the necessary equipment to fight the pandemic. Russia, however, then decided to send medical equipment to the United States rather than Kyrgyzstan. The Russians explained that the equipment was sent to New York as part of the so-called ordinary humanitarian aid (which was excluded from the decision taken by the Commission), but representatives of the U.S. State Department have officially admitted that the Russian side was paid for the delivery (*Tydzień*, 2020). It is worth noting that the Russians also sent their equipment, as well as medical personnel to fight the pandemic, to other Western countries, such as Italy (Sakwa, 2020). The Russian authorities hoped that this attitude would win them the favor of some Western countries and thus make it easier to lift the sanctions imposed on Russia after the annexation of Crimea (Legucka, 2020).

On 31 March, the Eurasian Intergovernmental Council took a decision on food security. The member states were to temporarily refrain from exporting food products to other countries. Many analysts tend to share the view that this decision was de facto a replication of the decisions of individual Member States by the Community. This can be seen very clearly when we look at the actions of the Russian government on the issue. In mid-March, the Russian authorities banned the sale of processed cereal products to other countries. A very similar decision was taken a few days later by Kazakhstan. Importantly, these decisions were taken without taking into account the difficult grain situation in two other Community members. Armenia and Kyrgyzstan are both countries with insufficient resources in this area and they have to rely on supplies from abroad. Armenia is able to meet (from its own resources) one-third of its total grain demand, Kyrgyzstan about a half.

The Russian Federation has taken (and continues to take) some actions to assist the countries in the post-Soviet space in their fight against coronavirus within the framework of bilateral relations. An example of this was the decision on 12 March 2020 to send 100,000 COVID-19 tests to 13 countries. They included Armenia, Azerbaijan, Belarus, Kazakhstan, Tajikistan, and Turkmenistan. It was a very important initiative as it made it possible to detect more virus cases in those countries. This assistance, however, was provided not within the Eurasian Economic Union, but in the framework of bilateral relations and was mainly aimed at strengthening Russia's position and influence in the post-Soviet space.

Another step (which is in line with the Russian strategy of basing foreign policy on bilateral relations) was the offer of assistance extended to Kazakhstan. In early July, Russian Prime Minister Mikhail Mishustin expressed readiness to provide support to Kazakhstan in its fight against coronavirus during a phone call with the head of the Kazakh government, Askar Mamin. The Kazakh side reported that the Russians were ready to send coronavirus tests, medicines, and experts who could help build infectious disease hospitals (*Kazachstan*, 2020).

The response of the countries making up the Eurasian Economic Union to the COVID-19 pandemic

The low effectiveness of the Eurasian Economic Union's efforts to combat the pandemic has prompted individual member states to develop ways to fight the coronavirus at national levels (Karaganov, Suslov, 2020). The following overview is a compilation of the most important decisions taken in the first and second phases of the pandemic in 2020 in Armenia, Belarus, Kazakhstan, Kyrgyzstan, and the Russian Federation itself.

By early January 2021, 162,000 people in Armenia had contracted COVID-19. The total death toll of the pandemic in the first month of the new year was 2,929 people. The first case of death caused by the virus was reported on 26 March 2020. Armenia has been more severely affected by coronavirus than Georgia and Azerbaijan. This is evident when looking at the number of those infected relative to the total population of all the three South Caucasus countries (Górecki, 2020). The most difficult epidemiological situation was seen in October and November 2020, when record increases in new coronavirus cases were registered. The highest daily number of new infections was recorded on 7 November, when 2,476 people contracted COVID-19 on a single day.

A nationwide state of emergency was imposed in Armenia from 16 March. The decision was taken after lengthy consultations between the government and other state institutions. The introduction of the state of emergency led to the suspension of a campaign related to a constitutional referendum that was to be held in May (Legieć, 2020b). The entire response to the coronavirus outbreak was coordinated by a specially created office of the Commandant. In order to contain the spread of the virus, both under the state of emergency and in earlier actions, the government of Nikola Pashinyan opted for a number of restrictions. A decision was taken to close the borders in the north and south of the country (with Georgia and Iran) to passenger traffic. Air links were also suspended. During the first wave of the pandemic, significant restrictions were also placed on gatherings. The organization of various events attended by more than 20 people was banned. Educational facilities and shopping malls were closed. Only grocery shops, pharmacies, and banks remained open. All public transport was suspended except for trains. There were also restrictions on leaving home. Traffic in the streets was monitored and anyone wishing to leave their home was required to have a specially completed form where they had to provide their home address and the reason for leaving home. Seniors (people over 65) could do shopping between 10 a.m. and 12 a.m. Importantly, the restrictions also applied to the religious sphere. All services in churches were held without the participation of people. This decision was also supported by the Catholicos of All Armenians Garegin II. Cinemas, pubs, sports facilities also remained closed. A remote education program was launched as well. Since the introduction of the state of emergency, lessons were broadcast on public television (*Koronawirus: aktualna*, 2020).

The Belarussian authorities did not take any action against the COVID-19 pandemic for a long time. Although the first case of infection with the virus was reported in Belarus as early as 27 February 2020, Alexander Lukashenko consistently downplayed the threat. In many statements, he claimed that the actions taken by other European countries were the result of excessive panic, to which he himself had no intention of succumbing. During the first wave of the pandemic, there was also no decision to close the borders (Kłysiński, 2020). These actions were intentional as there were fears that freezing of different economic sectors could lead to an economic failure of the state. It was predicted that an economic collapse would lead to massive social protests that could depose Alexander Lukashenko. Therefore, in the first months of the pandemic, neither schools nor shops were closed (*Białoruś*, 2020). Even sports competitions were not suspended, the best example of which was that first division football matches were played at a time when games were suspended across Europe. As more and more new cases emerged, the authorities recommended social distancing and encouraged the elderly to stay at their homes. Some minor restrictions were also imposed in gastronomy but they did not involve a shutdown of the industry (restaurateurs were advised to maintain 1.5-meter distances between tables). The adoption of such a strategy to fight coronavirus also resulted from the political calculation. Lukashenko, facing presidential elections just a few months away, decided to project the image of a politician who is in control of the epidemic and brings the number of new infections down (Kłysiński, 2020). This attitude of the Belarusian authorities greatly alarmed the World Health Organization. On 21 April, it appealed to the government in Minsk to cancel all mass events in the country and also to introduce a system of remote learning and certain restrictions on the movement of people. This would apply to people included in high-risk groups. The WHO also noticed that the regime of Alexander Lukashenko was deliberately not telling the population about the threat, so the appeal explicitly stated that the Belarusian authorities should transparently and regularly inform the public about the scale of the pandemic. However, all these instructions and recommendations were ignored by the Belarusian authorities, which led to a situation where the pandemic was no longer under control (*Białoruś*, 2020). While during the first wave (in April and May), according to official data, the daily rise in infections ranged between 800–1,000 people, by the end of the year the numbers were in the range of 1,700–1,940 people. By January 2021, 222,000 people had been infected with coronavirus in Belarus, 1,564 of whom had died. These are merely official figures, so the real scale of infections, as well as deaths, is certainly much greater. It is worth pointing out, however, that Alexander Lukashenko insists all these deaths are not caused by the coronavirus, but by underlying diseases in infected people. This attitude of the Belarusian authorities, along with the spread of information about the pandemic on internet portals and in social media, led to great discontent among many social groups (Kłysiński, Żochowski, 2020). This factor played an extremely important role in the mass protests that took place following the official results of the presidential election in Belarus in August 2020 (Żochowski, 2020).

The first coronavirus cases in Kazakhstan were reported on 13 March 2020 (*Kazachstan: pracownicy*, 2020). Kazakhstan was also the first country (of all the Central Asian republics) to report a death resulting from infection (this occurred on 28 March 2020) (*Pierwsza*, 2020). By early January 2021, 215,000 infections and 2,887 deaths had been reported in Kazakhstan. The scale of infections and casualties of the epidemic has certainly been (and still is) much greater because, in the first months of the pandemic, the official statistics (like in Kyrgyzstan) did not include people who were ill and died from pneumonia. It was only from 1 August that statistics began to link new coronavirus infections and pneumonia (*Epidemia*, 2020). A state of emergency was imposed in Kazakhstan due to the coronavirus outbreak on 16 March 2020. While it was in effect (until 11 May), shopping centers were closed, remote learning was in place and mass events could not be held in the country. From 28 March, people could leave their homes only to go shopping or go to work (*Pierwsza*, 2020). It is worth noting, however, that once the state of emergency was lifted, almost all the restrictions ceased to apply. This led to Kazakhstan having to deal with a second wave of the epidemic as early as June (*Kazachstan powraca*, 2020). Spikes in coronavirus infections were seen almost every day. For example, almost 2,000 new cases were reported on 9 July, while in June the daily increase fluctuated between 300 and 600 cases. It was then that President Kassym-Jomart Tokayev instructed the State Commission for the Prevention and Control of Coronavirus Infections to create (in a very short time) a plan of restrictions modeled on those introduced during the first lockdown. Importantly, according to Tokayev, the surging numbers of infections were caused by the irresponsible behavior of the citizens themselves, who did not maintain social distance. The new-old restrictions, which were introduced at the beginning of July, mainly affected the transport sector (the use of public transport between regions was banned, transport in cities was also restricted) and services (e.g. beauty salons, hairdressing salons, gyms, fitness clubs, swimming pools were closed). Residents of Kazakhstan were also banned from using beaches, water parks, and cultural institutions (such as museums).

The first three cases in Kyrgyzstan were reported on 18 March 2020, after people returned from a pilgrimage to Saudi Arabia. Interestingly, the first official death resulting from coronavirus infection was reported on 2 April 2020. By early January 2021, according to official data, there had been just over 83,000 cases and slightly more than 1,300 deaths in Kyrgyzstan. These are certainly underreported figures, which was in a way confirmed by a report of the inter-ministerial Commission for the Study of Humanitarian Assistance Distribution. The report found that the Ministry of Health deliberately underreported statistics showing the scale of the pandemic in the country. This was particularly true for the number of deaths caused by COVID-19 among medical personnel (*Kirgistan*, 2021). Importantly, the Ministry of Health did not include deaths caused by pneumonia when it compiled statistics on pandemic fatalities in 2020 (*Ukryta*, 2020). The Kyrgyz authorities took the first decisions to limit virus transmission within the country as early as mid-March. On 16 March, all schools, as well as universities, were closed and a day later mass gatherings attended by more than 50 people were banned. On 19 March, a decision was also taken to temporarily close the country's borders (Временный, 2020). A country-wide state of emergency was imposed in Kyrgyzstan during the first wave of the pandemic. On 24 March 2020, President Sooronbay Jeenbekov submitted to the Supreme Council a law on the introduction of a state of emergency in several cities (Bishkek, Osh, and Jalalabad) and three districts, which (originally) was to continue until 15 April (B, 2020). In Bishkek, a curfew was instituted (from 20:00 to 7:00) and significant restrictions were placed on the movement of people (*Koronawirus w*, 2020). It was forbidden to move around the capital by private transport (this restriction did not apply to people going to workplaces included on a special list created by the Bishkek police chief). At the end of March, a decision was taken on remote teaching in Kyrgyzstan. From 8 April, it was to take place via two TV channels (separately for children in grades 1–4 and pre-schoolers, and students in grades 5–11). More than 200 teachers were involved in remote teaching in two languages, Russian and Kyrgyz (Билим, 2020). The COVID-19 pandemic also left a significant mark on the political life of Kyrgyzstan. Already in April, two members of the government (the Deputy Prime Minister and the Minister of Health) were dismissed from their posts on the grounds that they had created a situation where coronavirus had spread all over the country (Вице-премьер-министр, 2020). In the autumn of 2020, parliamentary elections were held in Kyrgyzstan, after which public protests broke out, leading to the resignation of incumbent President Sooronbay Jeenbekov. The power, by a temporary decision of the parliament, was handed over to opposition politician Sadyr Japarov who had been released from prison (Marszewski, 2021).

The first two coronavirus cases in Russia were already reported in late January 2020 and these were two people coming from China. From March, the epidemic began to spread across the country at a very rapid pace. This was due to a number of external and internal factors. At the beginning of the epidemic, Russians returning from European countries (such as Germany or Italy) certainly contributed to the rising number of cases, while in the following months a huge role in this regard was played by a failure to maintain social distance (Legucka, 2020). Moreover, an inefficient health service, especially in the Russian countryside, has been (and still is)a significant problem in the fight against the pandemic. Analyzing the spread of the virus in the Russian Federation, it is easy to notice that from mid-March, in just 10 days, the number of infected people increased tenfold (from 63 to 658). This was partly caused by Russians returning to the country from epidemic-stricken Western European countries. At the end of 2020, the pandemic accelerated even more (Rogoża, 2020). December proved to be a particularly difficult month, with record increases in new cases. The highest number was recorded on 24 December, when almost 30,000 new COVID-19 cases emerged.

Despite the large increase in the number of ill people, restrictions related to the COVID-19 pandemic were introduced gradually and quite slowly in Russia. The first measures to stop virus transmission involved isolating people who were arriving from countries heavily affected by the pandemic in February 2020. In particular, efforts were made to isolate people who had been to China, Iran, and also European countries. The next step was a decision to close Russia's borders to foreigners. An appeal was made to Russian citizens to avoid large gatherings and reduce trips out of their homes. Only on 16 March did the authorities decide to close cultural institutions (such as museums and theatres) (Wiśniewska, 2020). Another example of the slow introduction of restrictions was in the field of education. The decision to close schools was taken only 52 days after the first COVID-19 case was reported. Compared to other (especially European) countries, this decision came relatively late. However, in an effort to contain the spread of the pandemic, the Russian authorities paid salaries to citizens even though public holidays had been declared (until the end of April 2020). It was also decided that it would be up to individual regions to determine the scale of restrictions on citizens. As it later turned out, during the first wave of the pandemic, complete self-isolation was mandated in 80 of the 85 entities that make up the Russian Federation. This meant that senior citizens (people over 65) were not allowed to go outside and other people had to stay within 100 meters of their homes. Compliance with these restrictions was enforced by a number of Russian services, including the National Guard and OMON (Benedyczak, 2020). In late March 2020, the State Duma passed a law that imposed heavy penalties for violations of sanitary rules. Anyone afflicted by COVID-19 who, through their irresponsible behavior, would infect a large number of people, could be fined up to one million roubles or sent to prison for three years. If one person died as a result of such an infection, the coronavirus "spreader" would face five years in prison, and in a situation where two people died, they would face up to seven years in a penal colony (Kułakowski, 2020). The Russian Federation was the first country to officially announce that a vaccine against coronavirus had been developed. The Russian President announced it back in early August and it was officially registered on 11 August 2020. After the United States, China, and the United Kingdom, Russia was the next country to join in an international competition of sorts to see who would be the first to achieve success in this field. It was believed that the development of a vaccine could yield many benefits, not only economic but also political. It is also worth noting that all the research in this area in the Russian Federation was carried out primarily by state institutes rather than private medical corporations (Benedyczak, Zaręba, 2020). In the context of international relations, in turn, an important role was played by disinformation campaigns that the Russian Federation has conducted (and still conducts). A good example of this was the dissemination of misinformation about an alleged blockade organized by Poland to obstruct the flight of a plane carrying medical aid to Italy. Such actions are of course part of the broader context of Russian policy, an essential element of which is to undermine the solidarity of the European Union countries (Legucka, Przychodniak, 2020).

Conclusion

Analyzing international relations in the Eurasian area, as well as internal processes in the former Soviet states during the COVID-19 pandemic, several conclusions can be drawn. The pandemic has shown that the integration structures which were created in the region at the initiative of the Russian Federation are incapable of effectively countering dangers such as biological threats. This is largely due to the fact that the foreign policy of the Russian Federation is focused on bilateral relations rather than on developing mechanisms that would take into account the interests of other countries belonging to international organizations operating in the area (such as the Eurasian Economic Union). The COVID-19 pandemic has also demonstrated that all the post-Soviet states are struggling with systemic health care inefficiencies. This is largely a result of insufficient financial resources. In each country in the region, statistics have been manipulated to hide the true scale of the pandemic. And this has posed (and will continue to pose) a certain threat to their internal stability. The numerous public protests that were organized in Belarus and Kyrgyzstan in 2020 are the best example here. The COVID-19 epidemic should therefore contribute (at least in theory) to a change in the thinking of the ruling elites with regard to increasing spending in the medical domain (Sanaei, 2020). What is equally important, the pandemic has shown that measures to combat coronavirus in the countries that make up the Eurasian Economic Union have been developed primarily at national levels.

References

Benedyczak J. (2020), *Przymus i kontrola – Rosja w trakcie epidemii COVID-19*, https://www.pism.pl/publikacje/Przymus_i_kontrola__Rosja_w_trakcie_epidemii_COVID19, (Accessed: 03.01.2021).

Benedyczak J., Zaręba Sz. (2020), *Międzynarodowy wyścig po szczepionkę na COVID-19*, https://www.pism.pl/publikacje/Miedzynarodowy_wyscig_po_szczepionke_na_COVID19, (Accessed: 06.01.2021).

Białoruś wobec COVID-19 – bezradność i bezczynność(2020), https://ies.lublin.pl/komentarze/bialorus-wobec-covid-19-bezradnosc-i-bezczynnosc/, (Accessed: 04.01.2021).

Билим берүү жана илим министрлиги видеосабактарды тартууну улантып жатат (2020), https://edu.gov.kg/kg/news/ministerstvo-obrazovaniya-i-nauki-prodolzhaet-snimat-videouroki/, (Accessed: 05.01.2021).

Epidemia koronawirusa. Kazachstan przedłuża ograniczenia związane z walką z Covid-19(2020), https://forsal.pl/swiat/aktualnosci/artykuly/7776590,epidemia-koronawirusa-kazachstan-przedluza-ograniczenia-zwiazane-z-walka-z-covid-19.html, (Accessed: 05.01.2021).

Górecki W. (2020), *Armenia: atak władz na oligarchę Carukiana*, https://www.osw.waw.pl/pl/publikacje/analizy/2020–06–17/armenia-atak-wladz-na-oligarche-carukiana, (Accessed: 29.12.2020).

Karaganov S., Suslov D. V. (2020), *Russia in the Post-Coronavirus World: New Ideas for Foreign Policy*, https://eng.globalaffairs.ru/articles/post-coronavirus-world/, (Accessed: 08.01.2021).

Kazachstan: pracownicy medyczni na pierwszej linii (2020), https://studium.uw.edu.pl/kazachstan-pracownicy-medyczni-na-pierwszej-linii/, (Accessed: 06.01.2021).

Kazachstan powraca do obostrzeń związanych z COVID-19 (2020), https://studium.uw.edu.pl/kazachstan-powraca-do-obostrzen-zwiazanych-z-covid-19/, (Accessed: 06.01.2021).

Kirgistan: skandal korupcyjny wokół COVID-19 (2021), https://studium.uw.edu.pl/kirgistan-skandal-korupcyjny-wokol-covid-19/, (Accessed: 05.01.2021).

Kłysiński K. (2020), *Białoruś wobec pandemii koronawirusa: zaprzeczanie faktom*, https://www.osw.waw.pl/pl/publikacje/analizy/2020–03–18/bialorus-wobec-pandemii-koronawirusa-zaprzeczanie-faktom, (Accessed: 04.01.2021).

Kłysiński K. Żochowski P., *Zaklinanie rzeczywistości: Białoruś w obliczu pandemii COVID-19*, https://www.osw.waw.pl/pl/publikacje/komentarze-osw/2020-04-03/zaklinanie-rzeczywistosci-bialorus-w-obliczu-pandemii-covid-19, (Accessed: 04.01.2021).

Koronawirus: aktualna sytuacja na Kaukazie Południowym (2020), https://studium.
uw.edu.pl/koronawirus-aktualna-sytuacja-na-kaukazie-poludniowym-10/, (Accessed: 27.12.2020).

Koronawirus w Kirgistanie: Stan wyjątkowy w trzech największych miastach w związku z Covid-19(2020), https://www.gazetaprawna.pl/wiadomosci/artykuly/1463218,koronawirus-kirgistan-stan-wyjatkowy-pandemia-covid-19.html, (Accessed: 05.01.2021).

Kułakowski T. (2020), *Koronawirus testuje Putina. „Wytoczy najcięższe działa"*, https://tvn24.pl/magazyn-tvn24/koronawirus-testuje-putina-wytoczy-najciezsze-dziala,265,4635, (Accessed: 05.01.2021).

Legieć A. (2020a), *Konsekwencje pandemii COVID-19 w Azji Centralnej*, https://www.pism.pl/publikacje/Konsekwencje_pandemii_COVID19_w_Azji_Centralnej, (Accessed: 04.01.2021).

Legieć A. (2020b), *Państwa Kaukazu Południowego wobec COVID-19*, https://www.pism.pl/publikacje/Panstwa_Kaukazu_Poludniowego_wobec_COVID19 (27.12.2020).

Legucka A. (2020), *Rosja wobec pandemii COVID-19*, https://pism.pl/publikacje/Rosja_wobec_pandemii_COVID19, (Accessed: 27.12.2020).

Legucka A., Przychodniak M. (2020), *Dezinformacja Chin i Rosji w trakcie pandemii COVID-19*, https://www.pism.pl/publikacje/Dezinformacja_Chin_i_Rosji_w_trakcie_pandemii_COVID19, (Accessed: 07.01.2021).

Marszewski M. (2021), *Kirgistan: zwycięstwo Dżaparowa i republiki prezydenckiej*, https://www.osw.waw.pl/pl/publikacje/analizy/2021–01–11/kirgistan-zwyciestwo-dzaparowa-i-republiki-prezydenckiej, (Accessed: 06.01.2021).

Обзор ключевых мер и решений ЕЭК (2020), http://www.eurasiancommission.org/ru/covid-19/Pages/measures.aspx, (Accessed: 05.01.2021).

Pierwsza śmiertelna ofiara COVID-19 w Azji Środkowej, https://studium.uw.edu.pl/pierwsza-smiertelna-ofiara-covid-19-w-azji-srodkowej/, (Accessed: 05.01.2021).

Radziwinowicz W. (2020), *COVID-19 w Rosji zabójczy jak wojna*, https://wyborcza.pl/7,75399,26603911,covid-19-w-rosji-zabojczy-jak-wojna.html, (Accessed: 14.01.2021).

Rogoża J. (2020), *Rosja: masowa akcja szczepień pod presją polityczną*, https://www.osw.waw.pl/pl/publikacje/analizy/2020–12–09/rosja-masowa-akcja-szczepien-pod-presja-polityczna, (Accessed: 27.12.2020).

Sakwa R. (2020), *Normality: Coronavirus and State Transformation*, https://eng.globalaffairs.ru/articles/normality-coronavirus/, (Accessed: 04.01.2021).

Sanaei M. (2020), *The World Order in the Post-Coronavirus Era*, https://eng.globalaffairs.ru/articles/world-order-post-corona/, (Accessed: 07.01.2021).

Tydzień w Azji: Rosja i Euroazjatycka Unia Gospodarcza – problemy w walce z koronawirusem (2020), https://instytutboyma.org/pl/tydzien-w-azji-problemy-na-bliskiej-zagranicy-rosja-i-euroazjatycka-unia-gospodarcza-w-walce-z-koronawirusem/, (Accessed: 27.12.2020).

Ukryta skala zagrożenia koronawirusem w Azji Środkowej (2020), https://studium.uw.edu.pl/ukryta-skala-zagrozenia-koronawirusem-w-azji-srodkowej/, (Accessed: 05.01.2021).

В Кыргызстане вводится режим чрезвычайного положения (2020), https://rus.azattyk.org/a/30505743.html, (Accessed: 05.01.2021).

Вице-премьер-министр Алтынай Омурбекова и министр здравоохранения Космосбек Чолпонбаев освобождены от должностей (2020), http://www.president.kg/ru/sobytiya/16431_vice_premer_ministr_altinay_omurbekova_iministr_zdravoohraneniya_kosmosbek_cholponbacv_osvoboghdeni_otdolgh-nostey, (Accessed: 05.01.2021).

Wiśniewska I. (2020), *Rosja wobec pandemii koronawirusa: pochwała oblężonej twierdzy*, https://www.osw.waw.pl/pl/publikacje/analizy/2020–03–18/rosja-wobec-pandemii-koronawirusa-pochwala-oblezonej-twierdzy, (Accessed: 05.01.2021).

Временный запрет на въезд иностранцев в Кыргызстан вводится с 19 марта (2020), https://www.vb.kg/doc/386252_vremennyy_zapret_na_vezd_inostrancev_v_kyrgyzstan_vvoditsia_s_19_marta.html/, (Accessed: 05.01.2021).

Żochowski P. (2020), *Białoruś na progu drugiego miesiąca protestów*, https://www.osw.waw.pl/pl/publikacje/analizy/2020–09–07/bialorus na progu-drugiego-miesiaca-protestow, (Accessed: 04.01.2021).

Zuzanna Pawłowska
Adam Mickiewicz University, Poznań
ORCID: 0000-0002-1817-4768
Jakub Rösler
Adam Mickiewicz University, Poznań
ORCID: 0000-0003-0672-7502
Julia Orłowska
Adam Mickiewicz University, Poznań
ORCID: 0000-0002-6021-1753

EUROPEAN HEALTH POLICY COOPERATION AND COMPETITION IN THE TIME OF THE COVID-19 PANDEMIC[1]

December 31, 2019 — it is on that exact day that the health commission in Wuhan, in the Chinese province of Hubei, officially announced new viral pneumonia cases. Initially, the news about the disease did not attract much public attention. In Poland, an article on this subject published in one of the national newspapers, *Rzeczpospolita*, was five times less popular than an entry about a woman who pulled Pope Francis by the hand (*China*, 2020). However, the world has significantly changed since December 31, 2019. Over a year, we gained a new perspective by verifying our previous beliefs about the degree of interdependence between countries. The scale of the problem, the rapid development of events, and the level of involvement of the international community, all proved that the COVID-19 pandemic a valuable experience on a global scale. The global focus on the problem has emerged not only due to the search for effective solutions but also due to the exposure of the weaknesses of modern systems. The COVID-19 pandemic brings

[1] The research was financed from the project „Research on COVID-19" from the funds of the Adam Mickiewicz University, Poznan

together the threats and challenges facing humanity in the twenty-first century. It is therefore only understandable that health policy and its effects are becoming a subject of interdisciplinary research, providing an overview of the changes caused by the coronavirus in the modern world — also in the field of international relations.

In just a few months, health has become a priority for nation-state governments. In early January, only a few cases of COVID-19 were known, on March, 7, the number of patients reached 100,000, and on April 4 — it exceeded 1,000,000. This means more than a tenfold increase in less than a month. The immediate reevaluation of domestic politics had consequences in international organizations that were put to the test in the face of danger. The coronavirus pandemic, due to its intensity and the multitude of areas it has affected, has become a rich field of research for international relations theorists. The threat has highlighted contemporary trends and has become a test of the quality of the partnership between various actors. This was particularly evident in the first months of the pandemic when national governments made decisions instinctively — not necessarily in line with their agreements and treaties. This was also the case with the members of the European Union, which is considered to be one of the most advanced integration projects today. The experiences of COVID-19 provoke reflection on changes in the contemporary order and on the planes on which they take place.

This work is an attempt to analyze the activities of the European Union and its members in the time of the COVID-19 pandemic, and the scope of the presented research covers the events from December 31, 2019, to January 1, 2021. Methods of institutional and legal analysis and system analysis had been for the research. The global epidemic threat led to a rapid increase in the role of health protection and health policy, which was reflected in contacts between states. The pandemic in this sector has highlighted the cooperation and competition between actors of international relations. We can notice it both in the relations of the European Union with external actors, in internal relations between the Member States, and even in the relations of the European Commission with members of the organization. It has become particularly visible on several levels: the use of non-pharmaceuticals, medical equipment and personnel, research activities, vaccines, and information activities. Our research aims to show the manifestations of cooperation and competition in these areas — to indicate their potential effects and to formulate recommendations. We ask ourselves about the framework of European cooperation in the field of health protection, with particular emphasis on its competences and attitudes adopted by individual actors.

As part of additional research, interviews were conducted with experts, analysts, and people professionally associated with the European Union: Piotr Kramarz, MD PhD, Filip Kaczmarek, prof., Jadwiga Kiwerska, prof., Bartłomiej Nowak, PhD, Lidia Gibadło, PhD, Tomasz Morozowski, PhD. The choice of the topic undertaken by us in this paper results indirectly from the reaction to the image of the European Union built in the first months of the COVID-19 pandemic. According to the report, „The image of the European Union in Poland during the first months of the COVID-19 pandemic," prepared by the Bronislaw Geremek Centre (Centrum im. prof. Bronisława Geremka), the attitude to the organization was negative and it echoed theories about the breakdown of EU structures. Our task is to contrast these opinions with reality, taking into account the actual course of events and analyzing the problem from the institutional side. The question concerns not only how the European Union and its Member States responded to the coronavirus pandemic, but also the extent to which these decisions could have been made. It turns out that the European Union has a small scope of competences in the field of health policy — which placed it in a less favorable position in operational terms in comparison to other actors. Member States were able to react on their own much faster and more flexibly, which resulted in an initial lack of coordination among the members of the organization. Our research, however, shows that the situation in terms of cooperation has stabilized after a few months, as well as the ineffectiveness of individualistic attitudes. The work also reveals a broader context of contemporary international relations, the changing coalitions of actors, and the balance of power. The coronavirus pandemic has become a catalyst, paradoxically accelerating globalization processes instead of slowing them down.

United in diversity? Analysis of the competences and activities of the European Union in the fight against the coronavirus. The institutional framework of the European Union

The coronavirus pandemic is not the first epidemic threat in the twenty-first century — although it is undoubtedly the first to affect Europe to such a large extent. Some researchers describe it as "the worst pandemic in 100 years" (*Fauci, 2020*), and medical journals go even as far as publishing studies comparing current events with the course of the Spanish flu of 1918 (Faust, Lin, Rio, 2020). Outbreaks of infectious diseases break out regularly, and the work of the centers dealing with their prevention and control is continuous. The emergence of a threat is usually influenced by random factors, which is why constant supervision plays an important role in this regard — experts from around the world monitor new outbreaks and conduct scientific research on this subject. Before the appearance of the coronavirus, there were indications that there was a risk of a global pandemic. Here, I shall use the information obtained during the interview with Piotr Kramarz, MD Ph.D., deputy chief scientist at the European Center for Disease Control and Prevention. He indicates that the first premise was the ever-closer interactions between humans and animals in food production and other processes, which increases the risk of zoonoses, which are infections that can pass from another species to a person. The second premise was globalization, and especially the development of international transport, which enables the transmission of the disease over long distances. In the interview, Kramarz admitted: "There were models that predicted a global pandemic to occur. They even pointed to Southeast Asia as a likely site of an outbreak, precisely because of the intensification of the practice of breeding animals for consumption on a very large scale" (interview with Kramarz, 2021).

The quoted statement shows that expert circles were aware of the existing risk. The main question was therefore not "will a worldwide pandemic break out?", but rather – "when will a worldwide pandemic break out?" — although this could not be estimated due to the randomness of infectious diseases. This is information that should be taken into account in the context of assessing the preparedness of the European Union and the Member States for COVID-19. Previous experiences with infectious diseases were regional or transregional (interview with Nowak, 2021). Although the effects of these events were incomparably smaller than that of the coronavirus, it allowed for the development of effective mechanisms and practices in the affected areas, as evidenced by the different course of the pandemic in Asia or Africa. Information on dealing with infectious diseases was therefore generally available and international organizations should be a repository of knowledge on this subject (interview with Nowak, 2021), but not every Member State has used it and had the experience in putting theory into practice. The European Union does not have a sufficiently developed set of instruments, and even if it did, the scope of the treaty's competences would make it impossible to use its full potential. There were no direct pandemic experiences that would provoke changes in the field of health protection. In support of this thesis, the 2009 A/H1N1v pandemic can be cited, as a result of which four important changes were introduced: 1) establishment of the Health Security Committee, 2) introduction of the idea of implementing joint purchases, 3) the concept of independence in terms of threat announcement and recommendations, 4) improvement in communication and information (Ryś, 2020). It was the first time in the history of the European Union that the Member States faced the threat of a pandemic on a large scale. This exposed the limitations of health organizations and gaps in the health systems of the Member States, allowing for improvements — but the experience was not so severe as to provoke revolutionary change.

The future may be different in the context of the coronavirus. For this purpose, the competencies of the organization should be analyzed. EU health policy has its origins in health and safety legislation. The competences of the European Union are defined in Art. 168 of the Treaty on the Functioning of the EU, from which we can read: "Union action, which shall complement national policies, shall be directed towards improving public health, preventing physical and mental illness and diseases, and obviating sources of danger to physical and mental health." At the very beginning, the scope of the European Union's competences has been clearly defined, them being only complementary and supportive. Member States make their own decisions and coordinate their own health policies and programs. Derogations occur in the case of food safety or the safety of medicinal products and medical devices. The organization's mandate in this context is greater than in the case of health policy. From the content of art. 168 shows that the activities of the European Union are limited to 1) supporting scientific research, 2) early warning, 3) creating platforms for cooperation, 4) monitoring threats, 5) prevention, 6) health education. Moreover, these competences are based on two dimensions: public health instruments and market instruments. Legislation on drugs and the manner of their circulation on the market is derived from articles on the common market of the European Union — the same is true for medical devices and tobacco (Ryś, 2020). However, there is no common health policy and the health systems of the Member States are very diverse. In fact, it is an area that is also influenced by other conditions — e.g. education, which plays an important role in the process of developing vaccination programs. In the field of health, the EU's competences are narrow, although improvements have been made to the system over the last years. The

2008 crisis has helped to look at state budgets and the labor market in this sector. Another important development occurred when patients started to submit complaints to the European Union for lack of access to health services, resulting in the creation of the "Directive of the European Parliament and of the Council on the application of patients' rights in cross-border healthcare" in 2011. In addition to codified rights for patients, it includes elements of cooperation between Member States (Ryś, 2020). As in the case of the 2009 pandemic, changes have been made, but the pace of transformation is not proportional to the increasing level of risk from communicable diseases.

In the institutional dimension, the European Commission plays a key role in the EU health care system, and within it the Commissioner for Health and Food Safety and its Directorate-General. There is also an early warning system for cross-border health threats, in which the coordinating function is performed by the Committee on Health Safety (Szymańska, 2020). Significant support for the European Commission is provided by the European Medicines Agency and the European Center for Disease Prevention and Control (ECDC). While the former employs almost 900 people, the latter employs only 300 workers. The coronavirus pandemic, however, has contributed to changes in this context, thanks to which both EU agencies will be enlarged and co-financed, as can already be seen in the funds allocated to them for their activities in 2021. Their work focuses on different fields and they have different responsibilities, but ultimately the goal of both is to ensure the safety of the citizens of the European Union. They often complement each other in their competences, as can be seen from the example of activities in the field of vaccination. The registration process itself, including the process of scientific evaluation of clinical trials, is the domain of the European Medicines Agency — in turn, ECDC deals with cooperation with advisory bodies of ministries and governments of the Member States in the field of building vaccination programs (interview with Kramarz, 2021).

It is also worth looking at the correspondence between the activities of the World Health Organization and the European Union, on the example of the activities of ECDC. We can see some gaps in the recommendations published by WHO and ECDC, e.g. in the context of safe distance in public spaces, although the agency's cooperation with the organization is close and intense. On the one hand, it is influenced by the aforementioned change introduced after the A / H1N1v pandemic, which determines greater independence in decision-making. At that time, this was due to the early declaration of a pandemic by WHO in 2009 and accusations of links with pharmaceutical companies which emerged as a response. On the other hand, the discrepancies in the wording of the recommendations were caused by the differences between the areas of activity of both centers. The natural partner of ECDC is the regional office in Copenhagen, but it covers over 50 countries and extends to the Pacific – this is due to the fact that after the collapse of the USSR, former Soviet bloc countries were included in its scope (interview with Kramarz, 2021). On the one hand, there are the countries of the European Union, and on the other, the Caucasus and Central Asia, which introduce a large variety of systems and economic situations. WHO recommendations must be adapted to these needs, assuming different technological advancements and circumstances. As a result, ECDC has to take a different position, often due to the conditions prevailing among the Member States. The geographical spread of the WHO European office in Copenhagen points to another important problem, especially in terms of the international competition and cooperation we will discuss later — it reveals the archaic nature and failure to adapt to the changing reality of multilateral institutions. In an interview given to us as part of the research, Dr. Bartłomiej Nowak states that: "COVID-19 has entered a period in international relations that is extremely difficult. He also found institutions that not only fell victim to the recourse to traditional mechanisms of power and self-interest but also those that are not reformed to deal effectively with the reality we have today." Many actors expected WHO to become the center of coordination for the pandemic, but this has proved impossible due to decades of weakness and fragmentation. The first thing results from the American-Chinese rivalry, which effectively blocks and undermines the organization's credibility, and the second — from the emergence of many important initiatives to fight pandemics outside the WHO structures, which affects its position in the context of international health protection (interview with Nowak, 2021).

Summarizing the analysis of the competences dimension and institutional framework of the European Union: it turns out that the integration project considered by many researchers to be one of the most complex international systems (Czachór, 2004: 24) has little potential in the field of health. This state of affairs results from the treaties regulating the functioning of the organization — which means that ground-breaking reforms in this area will not be introduced without changes at the same level. Meanwhile, treaty changes are a big step that most likely nobody will take in the coming years. The idea of health policy reform, including the recognition of public health as a competence shared by the European Union and the Member States, may face many obstacles: from the reluctance of decision-makers to the heterogeneity of health care systems (Szymańska, 2020). The prospect of treaty changes has not appeared in the EU's action program in the field of health for 2021–2027, and in the plans for the creation of the European Health Union, which only proposes a new regulation on serious cross-border threats to health and the strengthening of the European Medicines Agency and ECDC. This does not mean, however, that the road to reform is closed. During the interview, Dr. Bartłomiej Nowak stated that: "many reforms in the European Union, since the crisis of 2010, have taken place outside the treaties or in the shadow of the treaties. The European Stability Mechanism in the euro area was created through a separate treaty, that is, a separate international organization in general". The groundbreaking decision to issue Eurobonds, which was made in May 2020, also took place outside the treaties (interview with Nowak, 2020). Moreover, many of the positive actions of the European Union in the later phase of the pandemic, such as repatriation aid and vaccine negotiation, have proved that it is possible to work together effectively in the face of the current constraints. A practical solution may therefore be the creation of a new set of instruments or the development of good practices while maintaining the current competences in the treaties. Step-by-step approach Jean Monnet, one of the founding fathers of the community, developed his own concept of deepening cooperation on the continent and stated that "Europe will be forged in crises" (Sutowska, Polak, Skrzypek, 2017: 6). The theory of development through crises may become outdated due to the deterioration of risk management skills and an increase in susceptibility to external and internal attacks (Czachór, 2015: 10), but it is worth quoting and considering in the context of the coronavirus pandemic. There are many indications that the current events are not an existential crisis, and the decisions made by the members of the community and the European Commission prove that COVID-19 may become a catalyst for European integration. The current dimension of the EU's competences translated into international relations within the organization, increasing the competitive attitudes among the member states in the first months of the pandemic. The slow reaction of the European Commission, resulting from the impossibility of imposing solutions, gave nation-states free space to make uncoordinated decisions in the initial phase. This behavior has put the quality of the European partnership to the test and its effects can be felt for years. In addition, it resulted in many problems with the delivery of supplies and the flow of medical personnel, which additionally made it difficult to effectively fight the pandemic.

COVID-19 has brutally"reminded of the power of the state", which results directly from the constitution and mandates of national governments (interview with Kaczmarek, 2021). Natural mechanisms were visible even in the case of the actors most strongly involved in the development of the integration project. The decision made by the Federal Republic of Germany to ban exports and keep medical equipment on its market can be seen as a natural one — but that doesn't mean it was a good decision in the long run. The German government understood this and after two weeks it reflected on itself, but Italian citizens will remember their original attitude for a long time. The experiences of the pandemic have proved that in many areas an individualistic attitude does not pay off. The idea of improving the system may be increasing material reserves as well as improving and expanding the crisis coordination of the IPCR. The challenge for the European Union will be to build a community platform and mechanisms that will be able to inhibit the instinctive reactions of the Member States in the field of health protection. For politicians, voters and the society of their own country will always be the most important — so they must have proof that solidarity activities can provide them with more effective security and reduce losses.

Another lesson that can be drawn from the limited competences is the low visibility of the European Union and the inept emphasis on its own achievements. In the first months of the pandemic, public confidence in institutions was damaged. Healthcare achievements, such as financial support and strengthening the negotiating power of Member States in vaccine talks, have not risen in the media as loudly as the initial chaos and inaction. Moreover, politicians have often used the opportunity to appropriate the successes of an organization while blaming it for failures and delays. Ultimately, a small competency framework weakens the operational capabilities of the European Union in international relations. The area of health policy during the pandemic has become a field of clash of influence between actors. Limited opportunities, combined with a slower decision-making process put the organization in a more difficult position than state powers. This was particularly used by the People's Republic of China, which provided supplies of medical equipment to some Member States. On the one hand, it was taking advantage of the momentary weakness of the European Union and acting to undermine its authority, and on the other, it was an attempt to improve the image of China, still burdened by the outbreak of the Wuhan pandemic.

Cooperation and competition in the field of health policies

The COVID-19 pandemic has struck by surprise and influenced our reality on an unimaginable scale, affecting most of the spheres of life we know — from cultural events to politics and business. To understand the scale of the coronavirus's impact in the field of international relations, it is necessary to ask about the contemporary context, trends, and balance of power. Some of them were discussed in the previous chapter, and the first is the aforementioned crisis of multilateral institutions. The growing rivalry between the US and China weakens the most important and largest organizations in contemporary international relations. During the pandemic, it was especially visible in the case of the WHO and the United Nations, which, due to many years of weakening, were not able to react as effectively as they should. Quoting Małgorzata Bonikowska: "instead of a multilateral approach, we are heading towards the confrontation of two unilateral visions" (Bonikowska, 2020). The second factor is the changes in the balance of power. The emergence of significant actors in other parts of the world is slowly shifting the burden of power in international relations from the West to the East. Moreover, the lack of leadership, not to mention events such as the attack on the Capitol or difficulties in fighting the pandemic, all call for a reflection regarding the role of the United States (interview with Nowak, 2021). The third aspect is the growing importance of transnational actors. It was a recurrent topic during the pandemic, appearing in discussions about freedom of speech on the Internet and the role of corporations in the process of creating vaccines. This is also evident in the Covax initiative since it is made up of international organization, private companies, and non-governmental organizations such as the Bill & Melinda Gates Foundation and Global Alliance. Next to them are states (interview with Nowak, 2021). The last important thing is globalization. Contemporary threats are increasingly less of a regional nature, and the level of interdependence between actors is constantly deepening. The coronavirus pandemic has exposed the effects of these processes, as in the lens, highlighting threats on various levels, not only health protection. Some theorists have suggested that this may have an impact on the dynamics of this phenomenon in the future — but ask yourself whether it will slow down or accelerate due to illness.

Globalization has made today's international competition and cooperation much more multidimensional than in previous centuries. Various processes accelerating since the mid-1950s, combined with technological

development made it possible to transfer international contacts to new levels
— also to the area of health. According to the definition of the World Health
Organization, health policy "refers to decisions, plans, and actions that are
taken in order to achieve specific health policy goals in society". A clearly defined health policy, according to WHO, helps to build a vision of the future,
build understanding, inform the community, set priorities, and the role of
individual groups (*Health*, 2011). The American Centers for Disease Control and Prevention, in turn, in its definition focus on the legal dimension
— they indicate that "politics is laws, procedures, administrative actions, the
preventive or voluntary practice of governments and other institutions (...)
In the context of public health, policy development covers the development
and implementation of laws, regulations, or voluntary public health practices that influence system development, organizational change, and individual behavior to promote improved health". In line with these concepts, we
have defined five main areas on which international competition and cooperation in the field of health policy take place: 1) scientific activity, 2) non-
pharmaceutical agents, 3) medical equipment and personnel, 4) vaccines, 5)
information activities. In each of these areas, we can observe the increased
activity of international actors in 2020, and the actions taken in this area will
have an impact on their position in the post-pandemic period.

The first area that plays an important role not only during a pandemic but
also in its forecasting, is research. The exchange of information between experts plays an extremely important role in a crisis, although it is often over-
looked or underestimated in studies. Meanwhile, most decisions made in
the field of health policy have their source in the opinions of experts and the
exchange of experiences within this group. The European Medicines Agency, the European Medicines Center, and the European Centre for Disease
Prevention and Control play a leading role in this context in the European
Union., but we will focus on the activities of ECDC due to its nature, which
is closer to the subject of health policy. We can distinguish two main stages
of international cooperation in scientific exchange: the initial stage of the
pandemic, when we learned about the disease and measured the scale of the
threat, and the advanced stage of the pandemic, involving cooperation in
testing, treating the disease, looking for effective practices and vaccines. In
the European Union's view, it was important to exchange information with
Chinese scientists since the news of the new viral pneumonia appeared. The
exchange started in early January. Already years ago, ECDC has signed the
Memorandum of Understanding with the Chinese Center for Disease Con-

trol and Prevention, which is why the experts had a legal framework for cooperation and were in regular contact. Completeness of the information provided remains a contentious issue, as the Chinese partners are only an advisory body to the Chinese National Health Commission and probably did not always have the latest information (interview with Kramarz, 2021). We may suspect that the government of the People's Republic of China kept secret some of the data, but this is a difficult issue to quantify. In order to verify this, an international commission with access to sources and witnesses should be established (interview with Nowak, 2021). However, this will probably not happen due to the current position of China and the crisis of multilateral institutions. At the strictly expert level, however, there was a good flow of information, as evidenced by, for example, the rapid publication of the genetic sequence of the virus, which enabled the rapid development of vaccines. In addition to partners from China, throughout the pandemic, ECDC has been in contact with the European office of WHO, the American CDC, Africa CDC, with the countries of, so-called, „EU neighborhood" and many other foreign centers. Intensive cooperation in the field of research activities around the world allowed for faster solutions and intensified work on vaccines. It also allowed for the development of a common case definition which made it possible to reduce inaccuracies in the statistics. The very close cooperation between ECDC and the Member States should also be mentioned. Several groups of problems needed to be discussed among EU experts and specialists from the Member States: conducting tests, introducing restrictions, use of medical equipment, cross-border contacts, variants of the coronavirus. In the initial phase of the pandemic, if one of the countries was unable to detect cases, samples could be sent to the agency's laboratory network. There are also other positive effects of ECDC's cooperation with the Member States, such as the creation of platforms for the exchange of experiences, such as the NITAG Collaboration, or meetings within the framework of the ECDC Advisory Forum. Various anomalies can also be detected by exchanging information: for example, many Member States have proven to sequence less than 1% of virus isolates, causing problems in the detection of new disease variants. ECDC is now making an effort to allocate funds to help nation-state governments in this process (Interview with Kramarz, 2021). The coronavirus pandemic has exposed the power of globalization in terms of scientific experience — both inside and outside the European Union. In addition, collaboration is positively influenced by new telecommunications tools, enabling experts to stay in constant contact, build platforms and visit each other's sessions.

The second area in which we could observe the cooperation and competition of actors in international relations are non-pharmaceutical interventions — i.e. non-pharmaceutical measures also called restrictions. In the initial phase, the coronavirus pandemic triggered the natural responses of countries around the world in the form of closing borders and air connections. The impact of these activities was visible in the area of cross-border cooperation, having a particular impact on relations between the Member States. This is because governments made their own decisions about the movement of goods and people, although no one officially announced the abolition of the Schengen zone at the start of the pandemic. The uneven activities and the lack of cooperation within the European Union translated into the deterioration of the economic situation of individual members and hindered the provision of medical assistance to them. Many commercial contracts have been interrupted or disrupted due to a disrupted supply chain. It also contributed to declining in trust between European governments, an example of which is the May statements of the Italian minister of health, Roberto Speranza. He stated that "you cannot justify the attitude of some European countries that do not want to open borders to the inhabitants of Italy" (Wysocka, 2020). Travel difficulties also had a strong impact on tourism. In May, the Greek government decided to have passengers arriving from *high-risk* regions in Italy tested for the presence of the coronavirus. In case of the test being negative, the person was obliged to 7-day isolation, in the case of a positive test, a two-week quarantine was necessary. Veneto's head of government, Luca Zaia, commented at the time: "I wonder what the local tour operators think. Let them know that they will not see us again"(Wysocka, 2020). Such travel restriction events have taken place regularly. The Baltic states will remember for a long time the situation when Poland closed its borders and did not want to let them pass, which meant that many of them had to travel via a circuitous route (interview with Nowak, 2021). A positive reaction of the European Commission in the context of cross-border problems was the introduction of the so-called Green Corridors. Since March, their application by the Member States has been helping to maintain the smooth delivery of goods by allowing border crossings to be carried out in no more than 15 minutes. Earlier, e.g. on March 19, the queue at the Polish-German border was between 20 and 50 km long (Dorywalski, 2020). The closure of borders has also put people outside their homes and families living near the borders of the Member States in a difficult situation. In response to this problem, EU delegations, in cooperation with Member State embassies, coordinated the repatriation of over 650,000 EU citizens and helped cover the costs of over 400 joint repatriation flights organized by the Member States. However, public confidence has been undermined, and due to the low visibility of EU actions compared to the number of negative media messages, it has not been rebuilt. In the field of non-pharmaceuticals, the rivalry between the Member States was clearly visible at the start of the pandemic, during which each actor looked after their own interest. Positive phenomena, however, took place in the relationship between the Member States and the European Commission, and their cooperation helped to quickly improve the flow of people and goods within the European Union. The initial independent actions of the member states may have contributed to the weakening of the organization's position on the international stage, hitting its image as a united organism. The consequences of these actions could, however, make the governments of national states aware of the essence of cooperation and intermediation of the European Commission. In addition to restrictions on non-pharmaceutical measures, European cooperation played an important role: developing a testing strategy and using rapid antigen tests, mutual recognition of these tests, regulations regulating quarantine, cross-border contact tracing (*Pandemia*, 2021).

The third area of our consideration is the issue of medical equipment and personnel. The pandemic has led to a meteoric rise in the need for healthcare measures. Mass purchasing of masks, respirators, and protective equipment has begun. Among some Member States, the outbreak of the pandemic provoked protectionist reactions, an example of which was the aforementioned export ban introduced by Germany. However, it turned out to be ineffective and after some time such solutions were withdrawn. In the context of equipment and personnel, many solidarity activities within the European Union can be cited: 1) sending medical teams to other countries, 2) providing access to intensive care units to patients in critical condition, 3) sending air ambulance, pilots, and specialized personnel, 4) sending supplies medical supplies, 5) providing protective masks (*European*, 2021). The People's Republic of China also marked its presence in Europe in this area, which, although it provided less equipment than other EU countries, was able to plan it better in the context of public image (Jakóbowski, 2020). In the initial phase of the pandemic, when highly developed countries lacked resources in their respective markets, there was a race for medical equipment — in the advanced phase, when their own needs were met, the race for influence in countries worse coping with the disease began. Some people call this phenomenon"corona diplomacy". The rivalry of powers took place in many directions, it was particularly visible in the countries covered by the European Neighborhood Policy and in Africa. The following were active in providing aid: the European Union, the People's Republic of China, and the Russian Federation. In addition to the sheer scale of assistance in the provision of medical equipment, the quality of these deliveries also played an important role, which had a particular impact on the image of the Russian Federation. According to the PISM newsletter, US authorities sent back the respirators sent by the Russian Federation after they caught fire in hospitals in Russia, and the Italian newspaper *La Stampa* revealed that 80% of the masks it supplied were of poor quality. As a result, in June 41% of Italians were in favor of strengthening relations with the EU, while only 11% were in favor of closer cooperation with Russia (Legucka, 2020). The coronavirus pandemic is becoming a political test of the quality of partnership for many countries. The People's Republic of China gains the most, as it significantly strengthened its presence in Africa in 2020. China's role in this region has been very strong before, and COVID-19 may make it difficult to compete with its image in the future (interview with Kaczmarek, 2021). The European Union is in a worse position in this respect than national states because 1) it is composed of 27 members, which causes a blurring of merit, 2) it often acts through large UN agencies, e.g. World Food Program (interview with Kaczmarek, 2021). Moreover, the fact of China's visible presence in Europe and its assistance to member states proves that, as a result of the American-Chinese rivalry, Europe itself is becoming a battlefield for influence (Bonikowska, 2020). The coronavirus pandemic also prompted actors to reflect on the current state of international economic relations. This is the case due to, among others, safety concerns, as the production of key components of medical equipment was found to be concentrated in China during the pandemic. According to the Polish Economic Institute, this will induce states to withdraw production from the Middle Kingdom and accelerate the process of transferring the so-called "factories of the world" (*PIE*, 2020).

Another area in which competition and cooperation between actors in international relations became visible was the field of vaccines. This article is limited to the period 31 December 2019 to 1 January 2021, therefore we do not consider the process of implementing the programs itself and the difficulties encountered in delivering doses to the Member States. However, in the context of the European Union, there are two important spheres of activity in 2020: 1) participation in the vaccine race, 2) negotiations with medical concerns. The first is due to the potential benefits of prestige and profits for the winner, but also the willingness to contribute to the global effort to invent a cure. This is in line with the desire to make the European Union a force for positive solutions (interview with Nowak, 2021) and to create its own vector in the multipolar world (Bonikowska, 2021). The EU, together with WHO and other partners, organized an international conference in which it raised EUR 16 billion (EUR 1.4 billion from the EU) in commitments from international donors (*Covid-19*, 2021). The multilateral approach of the organization differs from the strategy chosen by the Russian Federation, which focuses on bilateral agreements, thanks to which it could strengthen relations with partners and generate more profits from sales. For this reason, Russia has also decided not to join the COVAX solidarity initiative promoted by WHO and international NGOs (Rogoża, Wiśniewska, 2020). In the case of China, the race in the production of COVID-19 vaccines is a matter of public image. In addition, the Chinese provided extensive aid in the form of loans in this area: African countries were reportedly promised to set aside $ 2 billion, while Latin America and the Caribbean were offered a loan of $ 1 billion to purchase vaccines (Brzozowska, 2020). Vaccines are important in the context of relations with third countries, but for the European Union, they were also important for internal reasons. The EU coordinated negotiations on behalf of all Member States and allocated EUR 2.15 billion for advance purchases from the Emergency Support Facility, a special EU mechanism introduced in response to the Covid-19 pandemic (*Covid-19*, 2021). In an interview conducted as part of our research, prof. Filip Kaczmarek stated that "the EU affects because of its scale. It gives negotiating power, also in talks of a commercial nature — it also shows the advantage of the EU and its Member States over developing or non-associated countries. They have neither that political power nor that negotiating power."

The last area where the influence of various actors in international relations visibly clashes is information activities. The media play an important role in the modern world, they are a space for image creation and help countries build their soft power. On the one hand, the European Union had to deal with the negative image forced in the news due to the defeat in the initial phase of the pandemic, and on the other hand, with disinformation spread against it by China and Russia. Moreover, in terms of health policy, an important factor is the way of communicating about the recommendations and the correct compliance with the restrictions. Meanwhile, many messages in this area are given in the wrong way, which affects the health of citizens — it is not enough just to put on a mask, you should also know how to wear it properly (interview with Kramarz, 2021). Difficulties in this regard have also been caused by the growing importance of conspiracy theories during a pandemic, often fueled by external actors such as China. This is important in ensuring the security of citizens of the European Union, as research has shown a link between belief in conspiracy theories and adherence to state restrictions (Allington, Dhavan, 2020). Adherence to government recommendations is one of the cornerstones of pandemic prevention and has a significant impact on disease transmission. The organization was faced with the consequences of activities in the information space in the social dimension, but they also had an impact on the EU's contacts with other actors. Serbia is a good example — during the pandemic, the Serbian government emphasized cooperation with China and the importance of its aid, although compared to the aid provided by the EU (approx. 800 million euro), Chinese support was smaller and mainly included the help of doctors and the construction of laboratories for testing (Przychodniak, 2020). However, this is an element of Serbia's pressure on the EU, reinforced by the narrative propagated (in Serbian) by a large number of social media accounts from the PRC (Przychodniak, 2020). A similar mechanism operated in some countries closely cooperating with the Russian Federation. The great influence of these countries and the level of their threat are because information activities are asymmetric. The European Union, based on civil values and liberties, cannot restrict freedom of speech and resort to the same practices as authoritarian states. The coronavirus pandemic has exposed the essence of security in this sector in contemporary international relations — it turns out that it doesn't only affect image but also indirectly affects public health.

References

Allington D., Dhavan N. (2020), *The relationship between conspiracy beliefs and compliance with public health guidance with regard to COVID-19*, Center for Countering Digital Hate, https://kclpure.kcl.ac.uk/portal/files/127048253/Allington_and_Dhavan_2020.pdf, (Accessed: 03.03.2021).

Bonikowska M. (2020), *Unia Europejska musi odnaleźć swoje miejsce w globalnej rywalizacji*, „Instytut Jagielloński", http://jagiellonski.pl/news/774/malgorzata_bonikowska_unia_europejska_musi_odnale_c_swoje_miejsce_w_globalnej_rywalizacji, (Accessed: 02.03.2021).

Bonikowska M., Kmiecicka J. (2020) *Po pandemii będą potrzebni liderzy łamiący schematy. Those acting in the "old way" will not count anymore*, "Wysokieobcasy.pl", https://www.wysokieobcasy.pl/wysokie-obcasy/7,158669,26144284,malgorza ta-bonikowska-po-koronawirusie-beda-pnecni-liderzy.html?disableRedirects= true, (Accessed: 03.03.2021).

Brzozowska E. (2020), *Co wiadomo o chińskiej szczepionce na koronawirusa?*, „Medonet.pl",https://www.medonet.pl/koronawirus-pytania-i-odpowiedzi/leczenie-koronawirusa,coronavac---chinska-szczepionka-na-covid-19,artykul,19126486. html, (Accessed: 03.03.2021).

Chiny: Najwcześniejszy zanotowany przypadek COVID-19 pochodzi z 17 listopada 2019 (2020), „Rzeczpospolita", https://www.rp.pl/Koronawirus-2019-nCoV/200319608-Chiny-Najwczesniejszy-zanotowany-przypadek-COVID-19-pochodzi-z-17-listopada-2019.html, data dostępu: 03.03.2021.

Czachór Z. (2004), *Zmiany i rozwój w systemie Unii Europejskiej po Traktacie z Maastricht*, Atla 2, Wrocław.

Czachór Z. (2015), *Kryzys w Unii Europejskiej. Propozycje nowych pól i pytań badawczych*, „Rocznik Integracji Europejskiej", No 9.

Dorywalski A. (2020), *Transport w czasie COVID-19, nowe zalecenia Komisji Europejskiej*, „Transport Logistyka Polska", https://tlp.org.pl/transport-w-czasie-covid-19-nowe-zalecenia-komisji-europejskiej/, (Accessed: 04.03.2021).

Europejska solidarność w praktyce (2021), https://www.consilium.europa.eu/pl/policies/coronavirus/european-solidarity-in-action/, (Accessed: 03.03.2021).

Faust J. S., Lin Z., del Rio C. (2020), *Comparison of Estimated Excess Deaths in New York City During the COVID-19 and 1918 Influenza Pandemics*, "JAMA" Netw Open, 3 (8).

Health system governance (2021), WHO, https://www.who.int/health-topics/health-systems-governance, (Accessed: 04.03.2021).

Legucka A. (2020), *Coronadiplication of Russia - assessment and prospects*, "PISM" https://www.pism.pl/publikacje/Koronadyawodacja_Rosji__ocena_i_perspektywy, (Accessed: 04.03.2021).

Nowak B. (2020), *Post-COVID multilateralism. How to save humanity from hell?*, Center for International Relations, https://csm.org.pl/analiza-csm-post-covid-multilateralism-how-to-save-humanity-from-hell/ (Accessed: 03.03.2021).

Pandemia Covid-19 i reakcja UE (2021), https://www.consilium.europa.eu/pl/policies/coronavirus/, (Accessed: 04.03.2021).

Piorun M. (2017) *Warszawa siedzibą Europejskiej Agencji Leków? Brexit szansą dla Polski*, „Radio Zet", https://zdrowie.radiozet.pl/Medycyna/Wiadomosci/Warszawa-po-Brexicie-moze-zostac-siedziba-Europejskiej-Agencji-Lekow,   (Accessed: 03.03.2021).

Polak A., Sutowski M., Skrzypek A. (2017), *Europa będzie się wykuwać w kryzysach? Scenariusze integracji w czasach polikryzysu*, Global Lab, Warszawa.

Prośniewski B., Bonikowska M. (2020), *Dr Małgorzata Bonikowska: koronawirus pokazał deficyty projektu europejskiego*, „Polskieradio24.pl", https://polskieradio24.pl/130/5925/Artykul/2503449,Dr-Malgorzata-Bonikowska-koronawirus-pokazal-deficyty-projektu-europejskiego, (Accessed: 03.03.2021).

Przychodniak M. (2020), *Znaczenie Bałkanów Zachodnich w polityce zagranicznej Chin*, PISM, https://www.pism.pl/publikacje/Znaczenie_Balkanow_Zachodnich__w_polityce_zagranicznej_Chin, (Accessed: 03.03.2021).

Rogoża J., Wiśniewska I. (2020) *Rosja w globalnym wyścigu szczepionek*, OSW https://www.osw.waw.pl/pl/publikacje/komentarze-osw/2020–10–28/rosja-w-globalnym-wyscigu-szczepionek, (Accessed: 03.03.2021).

Rosenthal M. (2020), *Fauci: COVID-19 Worst Pandemic in 100 years*, „Infectious Disease: Special Edition", https://www.idse.net/Covid-19/Article/10–20/Fauci--COVID-19-Worst-Pandemic-in-100-Years/60937#, (Accessed: 01.03.2021).

Ryś A., Bonikowska M. (2020), *CSM Live Meetings: What did EU institutions do in the first weeks of the pandemic?* Center for International Relations, https://www.facebook.com/153282818027787/videos/2772689406159634, (Accessed: 01.03.2021).

Schymalla I. (2020) *Andrzej Ryś: Co Unia Europejska robi w sprawie koronawirusa?*, „Medexpress", https://www.medexpress.pl/andrzej-rys-co-unia-europejska-robi-w-sprawie-koronawirusa/77203, (Accessed: 01.03.2021).

Sophie L. Vériter, Corneliu Bjolab, Joachim A. Koopsc (2020) *Tackling COVID-19 Disinformation: Internal and External Challenges for the European Union*, The Hague Journal of Diplomacy, No. 15 (4).

Sumisławska K. (2020), *Obraz Unii Europejskiej w Polsce w trakcie pierwszych miesięcy pandemii COVID-19*, Fundacja Centrum im. prof. Bronisława Geremka, Front Europejski.

Szymańska J. (2020), *Perspectives for the development of EU health policy after the COVID-19 pandemic*, "PISM", https://www.pism.pl/publikacje/Perspektywy_rozkieta_polityki_zdrowotnej_UE___po_pandemii_COVID19,   (Accessed: 03.03.2021).

Treaty on the Functioning of the European Union (2012) Official EN Journal of the European Union C 326/49

Tworzenie Europejskiej Unii Zdrowotnej: Większa gotowość i reagowanie na sytuacje kryzysowe w Europie (2021), https://ec.europa.eu/commission/presscorner/detail/pl/ip_20_2041, (Accessed: 03.03.2021).

Wysocka S. (2020) *Minister zdrowia: nieusprawiedliwione zamykanie granic przed Włochami*,   „Gazetaprawna.pl",   https://www.gazetaprawna.pl/wiadomosci/

artykuly/1480354,minister-zdrowia-nieusprawiedliwione-zamykanie-granic-przed-wlochami.html, (Accessed: 04.03.2021).

Zieleniewska M. (2020), *Pandemia COVID-19 może być równie tragiczna w skutkach, jak epidemia hiszpanki w 1918 roku*, „Medonet", https://www.medonet.pl/koronawirus/to-musisz-wiedziec,pandemia-covid-19-moze-byc-rownie-tragiczna-w-skutkach--jak-epidemia-hiszpanki-w-1918-roku,artykul,13221126.html, (Accessed: 02.03.2021).

Rafał Kamprowski
Adam Mickiewicz University, Poznan
https://orcid.org/0000-0002-9610-4394

RAW MATERIAL POLICY IN RARE-EARTH METALS AND HEALTH SECURITY DURING THE GLOBAL SARS-COV-2 PANDEMIC[1]

Introduction

The Sars-Cov-2 epidemic prevailing in Poland and in the world has shown how sensitive and fragile are national and international institutions responsible for creating security. The hard approach to security, dominating the political discourse for many years, and manifested by ever-greater investments in armaments or the development of strategic documents, turned out to be insufficient. An individual whose health, understood in accordance with the 1946 constitution of the World Health Organization, is the basis for achieving peace and security (Constitution of the World Health Organization, 1946). Politicians and scientists dealing with security must, taking into account contemporary realities, rediscover and define its health dimension, present in the 1994 Human Development Report. It is one of the foundations of the concept of human security, which aims to ensure a dignified life, survival, and development for people (Marczuk, 2014, p. 49).

The recognition of man as not only an object but also a subject of security, which we observe during the pandemic, follows with progressive technological development. As pope Francis pointed out in his encyclical Laudato Si, "technology has brought remedies to countless misfortunes that have

[1] The research was financed from the project „Research on COVID-19" from the funds of the Adam Mickiewicz University, Poznan

plagued and limited man" (Franciszek, 2015, p. 90). The miniaturization of devices that surrounds us and their increasing multi-functionality makes it easier for an individual to get to know the world around them. Technology that is developing exponentially is finally used in crisis situations, which we can undoubtedly include epidemics. During the Covid-19 pandemic, thanks to advanced technology, it is possible to monitor the temperature of the human body at a distance, and inform about contact with an infected person, or to use computer modeling and machine learning to better prepare for the next phases of the epidemic.

Rare-earth metals play one of the key roles in technological development, which is directly applicable in creating human health safety. They are used in the production of electronic devices such as televisions, computers, mobile phones, and the subject of the analysis in this article, respirators.

Raw material security as the main goal of the state's resource policy

Access to raw materials located in a given country has determined the level of its security for many decades. As noted by the leading representative of the realistic school of international relations, Hans Morgenthau, natural resources in the form of food or raw materials are the most durable components that contribute to the power of the state (Morgenthau, 1948, pp. 104–125). Kenneth Walz, in turn, adhering to the approach of structural realism, emphasized that the strength of the state results, inter alia, from the accumulation of such variables as the size of the population, territory, or natural resources (Waltz, 1979, p. 131).

Nowadays, the presence of resources in the area under state control does not translate directly into increasing its role as a resource power. The key factor enabling the above is having appropriately highly advanced technology influencing the possibility of their extraction, transport, and processing. The raw material policy is generally defined as geological research carried out by states – especially exploration and recognition of geological structures resources and possessed resources – and as their sharing through an appropriately developed transport and distribution network (Secomski, 1977, p. 204). It should be comprehensive, ie combine domestic and foreign investments with the exchange of experience and technical ideas. One of the main objectives of the raw materials policy is to support the development of the national and European economy by politicians by ensuring the security of raw materials (*Polityka surowcowa państwa*, 2018, p.5).

Raw material security, in contrast to the concept of resource policy, which was discussed by the authors, for example, in the interwar period, is a relatively new concept. In the European Union, the threats to the raw materials policy were noticed in 2008, when the Raw Materials Initiative was launched. It was guided by three goals: sustainable supply of raw materials from world markets, sustainable supply of raw materials in the European Union, and efficient resource management and supply of secondary raw materials through recycling (Komisja Europejska, 2008). In 2013, the Strategic Implementation Plan for the European Raw Materials Innovation Partnership was approved. Its main goal is to promote innovation in the overall chain of creating added value of raw materials by operating in the field of technological, non-technological, and international cooperation (Kudełko, Kulczycka, 2013, p. 237).

In Poland, the interest in raw material security, resulting in initiatives of a political nature, falls between the years 2011–2015. In that period, the Parliamentary Team of Raw Materials and Energy was active, whose aim was to create a framework for effective multidirectional development and to strengthen the position of the Republic of Poland based on its own natural resources and its energy source potential (Regulamin, 2015, § 1.). The results of the team's work became the basis for the appointment in 2016 of the Government Plenipotentiary for the State Raw Material Policy. Its main tasks include the coordination and initiation of activities in the field of the state's raw material policy or the development of new legal and economic solutions in the field of the state's raw material policy (Rada Ministrów, 2016, § 2.).

Raw material security is defined by all researchers as one of the basic factors shaping the economic security of the state (Płaczek, 2001, p. 140). For such a resource dimension of security, it becomes important to estimate the potential of the economic system of given countries to ensure access to raw materials from both domestic and foreign deposits. In the case of defining raw materials, the presence of which in a given area of the state is deficient, there is a need to guarantee stable and uninterrupted sources of supplies of this raw material from abroad. The security of raw materials also includes the strategic, key, and critical raw materials. Strategic and critical resources are indispensable in the event of a war. They are distinguished from each other mainly by the lower degree of their deficit in the economy of the state of war alert or the war economy (Misztal, 1974, p. 40). It is also worth noting that critical raw materials are difficult to obtain (Polityka Surowcowa Państwa, 2019). Nowadays, the group of strategic raw materials includes those compounds whose domestic extraction does not exceed 10%, thus unable to meet the needs. Key raw materials are, in turn, a group necessary for the proper functioning of the economy and satisfying the basic needs of the inhabitants (Bojanowicz, 2020).

Governments play an important role in the process of creating raw material security. They take place at the strategic level – taking into account the economic, political, and social situation at the level of the pre-investment phase (exploitation, extraction, and processing) and investment-related (cooperation with the private and local government sectors and non-governmental). Rare-earths play a special and increasingly important role in the raw materials policy due to the progressing technological development.

Rare-earth metals - characteristics and use

Although rare earth metals discovered mostly in the nineteenth century, only now are the subject of interest and political and economic game on an unprecedented scale, mainly between the largest powers, including the United States and the People's Republic of China. This group usually includes seventeen chemical elements: lanthanum, cerium, praseodymium, neodymium, promethium, samarium, europium, gadolinium, terbium, dysprosium, holmium, erbium, thulium, ytterbium, lutetium, scandium, and yttrium (Kamprowski, 2020, p. 112). Currently, they have become constant components of technological development, finding application in the construction of more and more advanced equipment. They have magnetic, catalytic, and luminescent properties (Gwynne, 2011, p. 3). Ever greater interest in the metals in question, both on the part of researchers and industry practitioners, has been observed since 1945. As Frank H. Speeding noted in one of the first articles comprehensively discussing this issue, the definition of metals as rare does not result from their small amount deposited in the ground, but from the difficulties in the process of their separation (Spedding, 1951, p. 26).

Rare-earth metals have many features that make them unique. The most important of them include high electrical conductivity, high gloss, and slight differences in their solubility and complexity (Voncken, 2016, p. 54). An important distinguishing feature is also significant resistance to high temperatures, without losing its plastic and resistance properties. Thanks to these properties, they are used primarily in modern technologies. They are used in the production of car catalysts, electric motors, permanent magnets, and optical filters. In addition, they are components used in the production of glass, ceramics, and in the metallurgical industry. Rare-earth metals are also used in medicine and biotechnology. Lanthanum carbonate plays a special role in these areas, as it has strong binding properties comparable to clay. Therefore,

Table 1. Date of discovery and modern use of rare-earth metals

Name of the metal	Use	Date of discovery
Scandium	Aircraft construction, mercury lamps, radiation therapy.	1879 r.
Lanthanum	Hybrid drive vehicles, optical glasses.	1839 r.
Yttrium	Catalysts, X-ray, cathode ray tube construction.	1789 r.
Cerium	Sparkling stones in lighters, metallurgy (as a deoxidizer), porcelain (as dyes).	1803 r.
Praseodymium	Catalysts, glass and porcelain coloring, metallurgical industry.	1885 r.
Neodymium	Laser technique, magnetic materials, production of specialized glasses.	1885 r.
Samarium	Laser and maser technology, magnetic materials, catalysts, nuclear technology, optical glasses.	1879 r.
Europium	Catalysts, rod construction in nuclear reactors.	1896 r.
Gadolinium	Nuclear technology, metallurgy, microwave technology, electronics industry.	1880 r.
Promethium	Isotope thickness gauges, source of beta radiation.	1945 r.
Terbium	Magnetic materials, laser technology, photo, and light-emitting diodes.	1843 r.
Dysprosium	Nuclear reactors, laser devices, catalysts.	1886 r.
Holmium	Nuclear technology, ferromagnetic and superconducting materials.	1878 r.
Erbium	Catalysts, dyes.	1843 r.
Thulium	Ferromagnetic materials, high-temperature superconductors, microelectronics.	1879 r.
Ytterbium	Production of aluminum and ferrites, catalysts.	1878 r.
Lutetium	Superconductors, ferrite production.	1907 r.

S o u r c e: own study.

it is used in the treatment of chronic kidney diseases and has a protective effect on the skeletal system (Zhang, Sun, Gu, et al., 2012, p. 90). The main application of the individual rare-earth metals is shown in the table 1.

There is a relatively small group of countries with the highest mining potential for rare-earths. They include China, the United States, Brazil, Sri Lanka, India, Australia. For many years, the United States had a dominant position in the rare-earth metals market. However, the situation has changed over the last twenty years, when they have become dependent on the import of valuable elements. It was related to, among others with much cheaper costs of their extraction and processing, with the simultaneous occurrence of significant domestic reserves. An important moment was also the closure of the American mines in Mountain Pass, from which most of the rare-earths came from until the mid-1990s. China took advantage of this situation and thanks to cheaper labor and the lack of effective regulations regarding environmental protection, the country has become the largest exporter of the metals in question. According to the U. S. Geological Survey, in 2020 China was responsible for nearly two-thirds of the world's production of rare-earth metals. They also have the largest deposits of these valuable elements on a global scale.

Chart 1. Global reserves of rare-earth metals by country

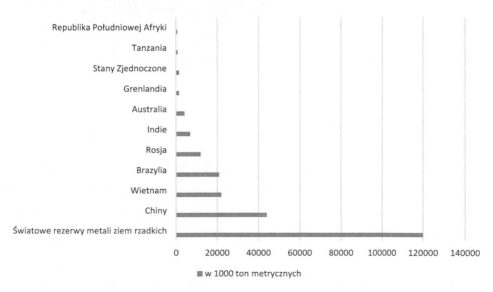

S o u r c e: own study, based on https://www.statista.com/statistics/277268/rare-earth-reserves-by-country/, access date: 02.03.2021.

Although China still has the largest deposits of rare-earth metals, in the recent period (especially since 2019), the United States is gradually regaining its significant position in the mining market of this group of metals. This is evidenced by the commissioning of the USA Rare Earth & Critical Minerals plant in Colorado. Its basic task will be to divide the obtained metals into three groups: heavy (dysprosium, terbium), medium, and light (neodymium, praseodymium). The investment commissioned in 2020 fully complied with the commercial policy of the former President of the United States, Donald Trump, consisting in making the supply chain independent of the elements critical for the American industry from the Chinese competitor (Trump, 2016, p. 53).

Chart 2. Extraction of rare-earth metals in 1994–2020, taking into account individual countries (in tonnes)

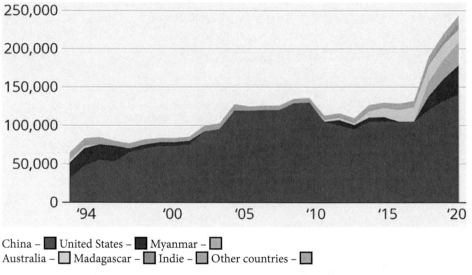

China – ▉ United States – ▉ Myanmar – ▉
Australia – ▢ Madagascar – ▉ Indie – ▉ Other countries – ▉

S o u r c e: own study, based on the United States Geological Survey 2020.

The balance of demand and supply in the global rare earth metals market has always been characterized by some instability (Charalampides, Vatalis, Apostoplos, Ploutarch-Nikolas, 2015, p. 131). The impact of the world Sars-Cov-2 pandemic in 2020 once again highlighted the difficulties in obtaining rare earth metals from outside China and highlighted the dependence on Chinese supplies for the rest of the country. While China maintains its dominant position in terms of both supply and demand for rare-earth metals, the increase in production of mines outside the country and the production of refined rare-earths is a key trend, required not only to meet the growing global demand but also to meet the changing demands of consumers.

The importance of rare earth metals in the aspect of the use of respirators enhancing health safety in the time of the Sars-Cov-2 pandemic

The pandemic, which quickly reached a global scale, was caused by the Sars-Cov-2 coronavirus. It initially began as an epidemic in the Chinese province of Wuhan on November 17, 2019. The World Health Organization was notified by China about the discovery of a new type of virus on December 31, 2019 (Scher, 2020). As a result of its transmission speed and health effects, the World Health Organization declared Covid-19 a pandemic on March 11, 2020. It then concluded that "the WHO assessed this epidemic around the clock and we are deeply concerned about both the alarming levels of spread and the severity of its effects... We, therefore, assessed that COVID-19 could be characterized as a pandemic" (WHO, 2020).

Progressive studies of the symptoms, course, and consequences of the disease have shown that, like other respiratory diseases, COVID-19 can cause permanent lung damage. COVID-19 pneumonia typically affects both lungs. The air sacs in the lungs fill with fluid, reducing their ability to absorb oxygen and causing shortness of breath, coughing, and other symptoms. In some people, breathing problems can become severe enough to require treatment in the hospital with oxygen or even a respirator to help circulate oxygen around the body (Cordis, 2020). This is the case when acute respiratory distress syndrome occurs. Access to unoccupied respirators played a particularly important role in the period before the development and implementation of mass vaccination against the Sars-Cov-2 virus. The chart below shows the number of free devices and the demand resulting from the rapidly growing number of patients.

In 2019, 77,000 new ventilators were enough to meet the global market demand. The situation changed drastically in 2020 when the United States alone needed more than 70,000 ventilators to cope with the growing number of hospitalized people. According to analysts related to GlobalData, in 2020 there was a need for about 880,000 new ventilators (GlobalData, 2020). There was also a noticeable increase in the seized devices in Poland. The crit-

Figure 3. The number of ventilators and additional number required in selected countries as of April 2020

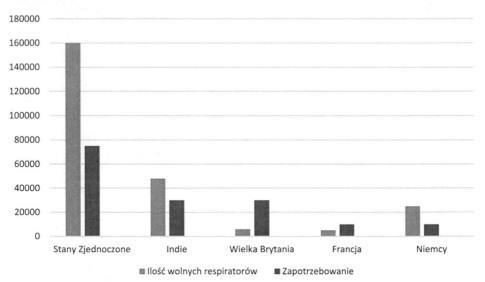

S o u r c e: own study, based on: https://www.statista.com/statistics/1122713/current-ventilators-and-additional-number-required-select-countries/, access date: 04/03/2021.

Chart 4. Number of occupied respirators in Poland in the period October 2020-March 2021

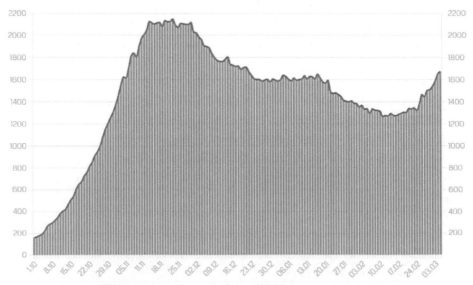

S o u r c e: Ministry of Health, https://www.medonet.pl/koronawirus/koronawirus-w-polsce,koronawirus-w-polsce--wrasta-lkieta-hospitalizacji-i-zajetych-respiratorow,artykul,58453053.html, access date: 05.03.2021.

ical moment was November 2020, when this number exceeded 2,000. The upward trend in the incidence since mid-February 2021 is also alarming.

In the pre-vaccination period, global demand for ventilators grew exponentially as the number of cases of Covid-19 increased. One of the most serious problems in the production of respirators was, and remains, the timely delivery of components due to the dependence on materials produced by global suppliers. The finished respirator is not manufactured from scratch. Individual countries specialize in the production of individual components of the device, thus creating networks of closely integrated suppliers of critical components, such as sensors or printed circuit boards. They are mainly produced in the United States, Japan, Germany, and Switzerland. A complete respirator consists of over 700 elements, which effectively extends the supply line of the device when the production of specific components is dispersed.

In 2018, the global ventilator market was valued at over one million dollars. In 2020, as a result of the spreading Covid-19 pandemic, it saw an in-

Fig. 1. Operation of the ventilator

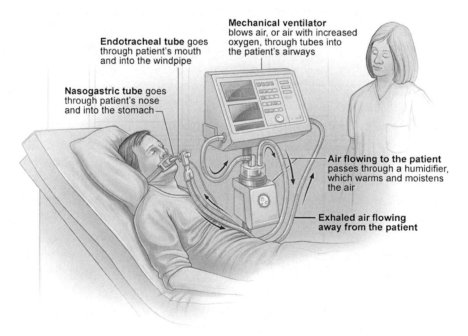

S o u r c e: https://www.nhlbi.nih.gov/health-topics/ventilatorventilator-support, access date: 05.03.2021.

crease of 172%. In the second half of 2020, healthcare companies increased their production pace to meet the high demand for these devices. Some of them, not related to the health industry, have decided to change their production line to support the supply of respirators. Another solution was to speed up product approval approvals to allow ventilator production volumes to be increased in a limited time frame. During the Covid-19 pandemic, the ventilator, as a device supporting or completely taking over the respiratory process, became, with the release of an effective vaccine on the market, the most desired device by all countries affected by the virus. The operation of the ventilator is illustrated in the graphic below.

Respirators currently operate by creating positive pressure in the lungs. They are divided into electric (they use energy obtained from energy networks) and pneumatic (they use energy stored in compressed gas). Modern technology enables the patient's breathing to be supported both in the treatment facility and at home (Wprost.pl, 2020). Rare-earth metals play an important role in the construction of medical devices. Particular attention should be paid to the use of the properties of tantalum. Its capacitive capabilities, as well as durability and high energy density, are the basis of advanced medical technologies such as respirators and life support monitoring equipment. High-performance ventilators rely on stable turbine control to synchronize the operation of the ventilator with the individual patient's breathing. Tantalum capacitors are located on the motor controller circuit board which helps to provide the desired speed control. Due to its high-temperature resistance properties, tantalum ensures stable and uninterrupted operation of the processor in a respirator.

Another element of respirators that use rare earth metals are magnetic assemblies. These are components that combine magnetic and non-magnetic materials in order to obtain a high magnetic field while reducing the cost of the device. Neodymium magnets replaced alnico and ferrite magnets. The electric motor of respirators is based on high-strength permanent magnets made of rare earth metals such as neodymium and praseodymium. The exhalation valve is an indispensable element of the device. The positive end expiratory pressure function can help patients retain some oxygen in the lungs and therefore extend the oxygenation time. Most current exhalation valves use a voice coil motor to drive a diaphragm to perform a linear displacement, and this displacement changes the throttle area in the fluid channel to dominate the on and off and flow rate so that inhalation and exhalation can be controlled. The respirator magnet is essentially a voice coil motor mag-

Fig. 2. Circuit board controlling the motor direction of the ventilator with tantalum capacitors

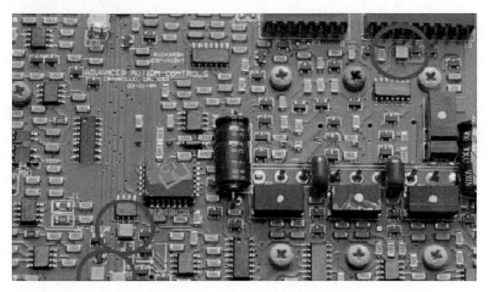

S o u r c e: Tantalum-Niobium International Study Center, "Bulletin", no. 181, April 2020, p. 4.

net. The current flowing through the coil is reflected from the magnets, thus creating inward and outward motion.

Summary

The global coronavirus pandemic has exposed and in some way exposed the weaknesses of the health security systems of individual countries. One of the more important factors contributing to this situation was and still is (albeit to a lesser extent) the availability of ventilators that support or replace the patient's muscles during respiratory work. In the construction of this device are used, among others. Rare-earth metals, which, thanks to their properties, contribute to a more stable and more efficient operation of respirators. Rare-earth metals are widely used in the production of other medical devices as well. The most famous types of medical equipment, which use rare earth metals are magnetic resonance imaging and computed tomography devices which are made of permanent magnetic materials. A factor that directly influences the construction of new respirators is certainly the fact that the production of components that make up this device is dispersed among individual countries. The pandemic is adding to the uncertainty resulting from extended delivery times. Some critical parts are only available in certain countries, such as Japan, Germany, or Switzerland. These countries, therefore, feel enormous pressure on their production capacities. The expected recovery of the global rare earth metal markets in 2021 may contribute to improving the supply of respirators. The key in this matter will be to secure the supply of permanent magnets and raw material for the production of life-saving respirators.

References

Adamas Intelligence. (2020), *New report: Rare Earth Magnet Market Outlook to 2030*, https://www.adamasintel.com/rare-earth-magnet-market-outlook-to-2030/, (Accessed: 04.03.2021).

Bojanowicz R. (2020), *Dźwignia rozwoju gospodarczego. Oto najważniejsze surowce dla przemysłu*, https://forsal.pl/biznes/przemysl/artykuly/8022875,surowce-kluczowe-strategiczne-krytyczne-lista-najwazniejszych-surowcow-dla-przemyslu-i-gospodarki.html, (Accessed: 28.02.2021).

Charalampides G., Vatalis Konstantinos, Apostoplos B., Ploutarch-Nikolas B. (2015), *Rare Earth Elements: Industrial Applications and Economic Dependency of Europe*, „Procedia Economics and Finance", vol. 24.

Cordis (2020), *Jak COVID-19 uszkadza płuca*, https://cordis.europa.eu/article/id/421597-how-covid-19-damages-the-lungs/pl, (Accessed: 02.03.2021).

Dias A., Bobba P., Carrara S., Plazzotta B. (2020), *The Role of Rare Eearth Elements in Wind Energy and Electric Mobility. An analysis of future supply/demand balances*, Luxemburg.

Franciszek. (2015), *Laudato Si*, Wrocław.

GlobalData (2020), *880,000 global ventilator shortage can only be met by new simple design requiring minimal operator training time*, https://www.globaldata.com/880000-global-ventilator-shortage-can-only-be-met-by-new-simple-design-requiring-minimal-operator-training-time-says-globaldata/, (Accessed: 04.03.2021).

Gwynne P. (2011), *Resuscitating the Rare Earths*, „Research Technology Management", vol. 54, no 3.

Kamprowski R. (2020), *Uwarunkowania surowcowe produkcji dronów*, w: *Wykorzystanie dronów i robotów w systemach bezpieczeństwa. Teoria i praktyka*, red. R. Kamprowski, M. Skarżyński, Poznań.

Komisja Europejska. (2008), *Policy and strategy for raw materials*, ec.europa.eu/growth/sectors/raw-materials/policy-strategy_en, (Accessed: 05. 03. 2021).

Konstytucja Światowej Organizacji Zdrowia (1946), Dz. U. 1948 nr 61 poz. 477.

Kudełko J., Kulczycka J. (2013), *Priorytetyzacja działań zaproponowanych w Strategicznym Planie Wdrażania Europejskiego Partnerstwa Innowacji w Dziedzinie Surowców z punktu widzenia polskiej gospodarki*, „Zeszyty naukowe Instytutu Gospodarki Surowcami Mineralnymi i Energią Polskiej Akademii Nauk", vol. 85.

Marczak K. (2014), *Pojęcie i zakresy human security*, w: *Trzy wymiary współczesnego bezpieczeństwa*, red. S. Sulowski, M. Brzeziński, Warszawa.

Misztal J. (1974), *Surowce strategiczne*, Warszawa.

Morgenthau H. J. (1948), *Politics Among Nations. The Struggle for Power and Peace*, New York.

Płaczek J. (2001), *Gospodarka obronna Polski w końcu lat dziewięćdziesiątych: szanse i zagrożenia*, Warszawa.

Polityka Surowcowa Państwa (2019), Surowce kluczowe, strategiczne i krytyczne, http://psp.mos.gov.pl/aktualnosci/66-surowce-kluczowe-strategiczne-i-krytyczne.html, (Accessed: 24.02.2021).

Polityka surowcowa państwa (2018), Warszawa.

Rada Ministrów (2016), *Rozporządzenie Rady Ministrów z dnia 9 maja 2016 r. w sprawie ustanowienia Pełnomocnika Rządu do spraw Polityki Surowcowej Państwa*.

Regulamin parlamentarnego zespołu surowców i energii (2015).

Scher I. (2020), *The first COVID-19 case originated on November 17, according to Chinese officials searching for 'patient zero'*, https://www.businessinsider.com/coronavirus-patients-zero-contracted-case-november-2020–3?IR=T, (Accessed: 04.03.2021).

Secomski K. (1977), *Polityka społeczno-ekonomiczna: zarys teorii*, Warszawa.

Spedding F. H. (1951), *The Rare Earths*, „Scientific American", vol. 185, no 5.

Trump D. (2016), *Donald Trump. Prezydent Biznesmen*, Warszawa.

Voncknen J. H. (2016), *The Rare Earth Elements. An Introduction*, Delft.

Waltz K. (1979), *Theory of International Politics*, New York.

WHO (2020), *Rolling updates on coronavirus disease (COVID-19)*, https://www.who.int/emergencies/diseases/novel-coronavirus-2019/events-as-they-happen, (Accessed: 03.03.2021)

Wprost.pl (2020), *Jak działa respirator?*, https://zdrowie.wprost.pl/koronawirus/10310402/jak-dziala-respirator.html?utm_source=zdrowie.wprost.pl&utm_medium=recommendation&utm_campaign=autoload-return, (Accessed: 03.03.2021)

Zhang J., Sun J., Gu G., Hao X., Wang S. (2012)., *Effects of La^{3+} on osteogenic and adipogenic differentiation of primary mouse bone marrow stromal cells*, „Journal of Rare Earths", vol. 30, no 1.

INTERVIEWS

Interview with prof. Robert Jervis, February 10ᵗʰ, 2021

Robert Jervis is Adlai E. Stevenson Professor of International Politics at Columbia University. His most recent book is *Why Intelligence Fails: Lessons from the Iranian Revolution and the Iraq War* (Cornell University Press, 2010). His book, *System Effects: Complexity in Political Life* (Princeton University Press, 1997) was a co-winner of the APSA's Psychology Section Best Book Award, and *The Meaning of the Nuclear Revolution* (Cornell University Press, 1989) won the Grawemeyer Award for Ideas Improving World Order. He is also the author of *The Logic of Images in International Relations* (Princeton University Press, 1970; 2d ed., Columbia University Press, 1989), *Perception and Misperception in International Politics* (Princeton University Press, 1976), *The Illogic of American Nuclear Strategy* (Cornell University Press, 1984), *American Foreign Policy in a New Era* (Routledge, 2005), and over 150 other publications.

Radosław Fiedler (RF): What is the legacy of Trump's foreign policy? What can and cannot be continued in the foreign policy of the Biden administration?

Robert Jervis (RJ): Bilateral trade balance, which really has very little meaning, so I do not think Biden will continue with that, but partly because it is changing in China, and I think Biden and his people, like Curt Campbell, realize that they cannot pick up where Obama left off and in some form, stiffer measures are needed, but probably for Biden, it will be at the broad strategic issues, rather than only trade. Biden, unlike Trump, would try to bring his allies in. In the Middle East, I think and hope Biden would build on the fact that some of Trump's policies enabled Israel to normalize relations with other countries. The biggest and the most important country is Saudi Arabia, and they are not yet ready to normalize relations, but there is progress made in the region and it is facilitated by Trump. In some small areas, Trump's policy may change. As part of the price for Morocco to recognize Israel, the US recognized its control over the disputed areas. The question has arisen – can we combine that with a more even-handed policy towards Palestinians, to make progress on peace or better relations or movement towards a two-state solution? That is very ambitious. I am not sure if that is true, but the other side of that coin of better relations of various Arab states with Israel and including Saudi Arabia. Moreover, Biden first wants to normalize and go back to JCPOA with Iran, he wants to build on that in various ways, but that runs in opposition not only for Israel but also from Saudi Arabia and others in the Persian Gulf, where Trumps had to strengthen relations. The questions for Biden is how do you continue better relations with Israel and the Gulf States and at the same time continue with Iranian policy and resuscitating JCPOA?

RF: There is some criticism from Bolton, Dubovitz, and others, who state in an open letter and advise against going back to JCPOA. The deal is outdated and it has to be changed, so which conditions should Iran fulfil? Iran declared that the USA should just lift the sanctions and return to recognizing the deal internationally. What is the road map for the US to re-join the deal?

RJ: It is a very bumpy road. You are absolutely right: several provisions expire pretty soon. One idea was not to look back at JCPOA and negotiate a new agreement. It is very hard and I think the new administration advised him wisely to first get back to JCPOA and then talk about extending and broadening it. Even though the Iranian economy is weak I do not think we can ask for too much unilaterally. Of course, getting back to JCPOA sounds quite easy, but as I will discuss with my class tomorrow there are enormous timing problems. Iran says: *You drop all your sanctions and we will drop the project*. Biden says, *No, no, no! You first come back to compliance*. The other problem is that Trump's people were quite clever in trying to limit the Biden administration. The number of sanctions that are in place at the moment, one of them is justified based on anti-terrorist statures. The Ones that are related to the nuclear side, Biden can weaver or lift by a stroke of the pen, but those others related to security need extra findings from the treasury department or maybe the intelligence community, so he cannot lift all the sanctions immediately even if he wanted to. And of course, there are domestic political problems as you know, on both sides. Presidential elections are coming up in Iran and JCPOA is not popular in Iran, since the economic benefits expected did not fully materialize, not mentioning American actions. On the American side, remember that JCPOA was opposed by the majority of Congress. It is not highly popular. The letter you referred to was open about it. I have to say it is very hypocritical for Bolton to say that Biden should behave in a bipartisan way, for him to say that... just give me a break. They opposed the JCPOA from the beginning so of course, they will oppose it now. Intellectually, I do not take it very seriously, but politically I say it is an indication that domestic politics here for Biden are not easy.

RF: Looking globally at US policy towards China, there is a substantial amount of Trump's legacy that will be continued. What about competition in different areas between the USA and China? Is it possible to avoid the Thucydides Trap? Can some peaceful coexistence be possible with Xi Jin Ping's style of leadership? Is there some room for accommodating China's leadership with Biden's policy?

RJ: I can only speak on the American side and I think there is room for the cooperation of two kinds. First, with the obvious global issues like fighting the pandemic, climate change, stabilizing world economy in which interest is not identical but there is a lot of overlap; second there are key strategic issues, in which there is conflict – China wants to push us entirely out of East Asia region, certainly it wants us to stop sailing our warships on what they consider their waters, and may want to build up a so-called wall of sand. It is not surprising, I mean under what theory of international policy do we expect a large country, which an especially glorious past and 100 years of weakness, which starts to recover, we do not expect such a country not to influence its region? We do not have to depict Xi as Hitler, or having some unusually aggressive intentions to adjust some relations as power relations changed. The question is what that adjustment is? And obviously for Xi and China a key issue in Taiwan. Ever since the normalization we were able to push that off to the future and say: "well if Taiwan wants to unify that's ok with us, we do not stand in a way of that, but coercion should not be used." Chinese leaders have been patient since they have believed that in the long run, things were going their way. Now maybe that belief is harder, looking at changes in Taiwan's domestic policies, and at what China is doing in Hong

Kong, we see that China cannot be trusted with "One country – two social systems". It's harder for Chinese leaders to think that things are moving in their direction in terms of Taiwan eventually joining. That is the most dangerous issue, hard to compromise. I think the current situation, where the US makes it clear to Taiwan that it cannot declare independence does a lot. It makes it clear that China if they engage militarily, or even blockade that will be very costly and risky. I think it can be maintained for at least four years but it is a tricky situation.

RF: Is the liberal paradigm still useful in analyzing the current situation and tendencies in IR? What about all the foreseen benefits of globalization that it promised, especially during the time of the pandemic?

RJ: Well, I think the heavily idealized view of globalization and total, uninhibited division of labour and also the political counterpart that this would lead to – good relations – that few mid-British liberals in the nineteenth century and also thinkers in Europe and US in 1920's proposed, was never right and always exaggerated. The pandemic and the right-wing backlash in Europe and the US made that clear. I do not think that we should, nor will abandon all of that. I mean extensive foreign trade has increased the wealth of all the countries enormously, but it is not done equitably but there is a consensus that we have to pay as much attention to the equity within the country and not to the pure increase of the GDP. It is a hard balance and easier said than done, but can be done in each country. Dani Roderick from Harvard Kennedy School talks about how you can craft trade in connection to the social contract within each country. There will always be friction, but I think we should not polarise and have completely uninhibited free trade or go back to the highly protectionist approach, where we can have a cake and eat it too? There are middle paths, where we have trade agreements and domestic policy instruments that can get many benefits. On medical supplies, countries may do more on-shore and be willing to pay more in peacetime (times of good health). We will see. People always say that in the time of crisis and then when the crisis has passed and they have to pay more to stock up masks or build the capacity for masks and medication they are unwilling to pay the price and go back to rely on low-cost producers.

RF: What advice do you have for Poland and Hungary, where we have seen some forms of authoritarian activity, such as suppressing sexual minorities, suppressing free media, and introducing many more limitations in connection to the Biden administration? Having in mind Navalny's

case, do you think having strong democracies in Poland and Hungary would be good for countering Russia? What should be done for better cooperation and atmosphere in general in Central Europe, especially in terms of Poland and Hungary with the Biden's administration?

RJ: I think first with Navalny and Russia, we see that Russia is a dictatorship. Biden will be much more consistent than Trump. Trump has had his policy, he followed, and then there was Pompeo and the rest of the government that followed their own. Within the Biden administration, there probably will be his policy with a public spotlight on the abuses and we will use our pressure, but we do not have that much leverage to go and say we are not going to do any arms control agreements as long as you are a dictatorship. Our leverage is limited and mostly funded on the belief to keep the spirit of democracy alive in Russia over the long run. Poland and Hungary, of course, it is different there. In Europe, they are in NATO and the EU. First of all, the break will be sharper, because as you know Trump was not critical towards authoritarian leaders, unlike Biden. I think not only that, but mostly he will work with other European countries. He feels that Europe should join to lead because of geographical, historical, and institutional connections. The US will not passively follow but engage with discussions with Europe on what the policies should be, we will listen carefully and try to make a joint policy. Europeans will be at the lead and the US will support that. Now the effect of that will be changing other countries' domestic atmosphere and domestic policies, but I think we will see the US doing much more itself and supporting the cooperation with the European allies.

The great contribution of Piotr Baranowski in transcribing of interview

Interview with Piotr Kramarz, February 3rd 2021.

Piotr Kramarz, MD., PhD., deputy chief scientist at the European Center for Disease Prevention and Control (ECDC).

Julia Orłowska (JO): Good afternoon. To begin with, I would like to go back to the period before the spread of COVID-19. Before that, there were events such as Ebola or the swine flu pandemic in 2009. Based on these previous experiences, can we say that we expected a worldwide pandemic to break out?

Piotr Kramarz (PK): Yes, there were such signals. Not even signals, but scientific studies have shown that there is a risk of this kind of pandemic. This was due to various global processes. One of them is the ever-closer interaction between humans and animals in food production and other processes, where there is a high risk of so-called zoonoses. These are infections that can pass from an animal to a person. Interspecies contacts appear to be intensifying and this risk is increasing. Historically speaking, such situations had probably taken place before, but they did not spread as quickly because the world was not connected to the same extent. The second process is globalization. The world got „smaller", and if there is a pathogen shift to the human species, it is spreading very quickly via international transport. This was seen in the 2009 flu pandemic and it is what we are observing right now, with the coronavirus pandemic. There have been models that predicted a global pandemic They even pointed to Southeast Asia as a likely site of an outbreak, precisely because of the intensification of very large-scale farming practices for human consumption and close contacts between people working on farms and in the various markets where live animals are sold. It looked as though something like this could happen there, but it was hard to tell when it would happen, as these are random events. However, we were preparing for this on the part of the ECDC, we have a whole range of activities, which are covered by the term "preparedness". As for the work of ECDC, for example, we have an emergency procedure, and if necessary, we activate it and switch to this mode of work. We have a schedule that defines the different functions, and we have two-week shifts, for example as public health emergency managers, when we coordinate the work of our Center in response to a public health incident such as a pandemic. So for the ECDC, this preparation had taken place and hasn't been only a procedure, because the procedures obviously need to be practiced, so we had simulation exercises, where we simulated incidents such as a pandemic and we practiced what actions should be taken not only at the ECDC but also concerning our external partners. That sums up the internal preparation of the ECDC. From the perspective of the European Union Member States, it seems, as far as we know, that at the beginning of the coronavirus pandemic all of the Member States had a pandemic preparedness plan. In general, it was prepared rather for a flu pandemic, but the coronavirus pandemic also falls under these categories of pandemic plans. Therefore, very early last year, around February or March, we encouraged countries to activate their pandemic plans. These obviously vary a lot depending on the health service structure in a given country and have been updated to a different degree. In some countries, they are relatively recent whereas, in others, they have been formed a bit earlier. Nevertheless, Member States activated these plans quite early in the pandemic. What hasn't been anticipated was the length of the COVID-19 pandemic. It's much longer than anything we've ever experienced before, once we've activated our emergency procedure. Usually, it was a maximum of three months, but now it has been going on for over a year — also the length exceeds everything that we previously predicted and we had to adapt our procedures and our work mode accordingly.

JO: How can we evaluate the initial flow of information regarding the coronavirus? Did information from China reach us immediately or, was the access to it limited? How did you cooperate with scientists from China and did such cooperation take place at all?

PK: At the expert level, such cooperation has been in place since the beginning of January last year, since we heard about the outbreak of atypical pneumonia in Wuhan. Our cooperation is based mainly on contacts with the Chinese CDC. We have signed the memorandum of understanding for years, which is why we had a legal basis for cooperation and we were in regular contact. We got information about what was going on. One problem was that in the early days of fighting the epidemic in China, the CDC was an advisory body to the National Health Commission and probably didn't always have the latest information to share. However, we had very good co-operation and colleagues from China shared information with us. They sent us reports, we had webinars and videoconferences with them, not only on epidemiological topics but there were also videoconferences with clinical experts who treated early cases of COVID-19 and shared their experiences with colleagues from Europe and the rest of the world. It was going very well. Another example of information sharing was the rapid publication of the genetic sequence of a virus, which made the fast development of the vaccines possible. On the other hand, the question of how complete was the information that was disclosed to us is difficult for me and anyone else to answer. On our part, on the expert level, the contacts were good and we received a lot of information, which we used on an ongoing basis in our work.

JO: What are the competences of the European Union in the field of health policy? There is, of course, the European Center for Prevention and Control of Diseases and the European Medicines Agency — however, when we talk about the competences of the EU in the field of health policy in general, are these competences sufficient?

PK: The mandate of the European Commission and agencies like ours in the field of public health is not very strong. According to the Treaty on the Functioning of the European Union, decisions on health protection and the functioning of the health care system are entirely the responsibility of the Member States. Our function as EU institutions, such as the European Commission or our agency, is to complement what countries do, help and coordinate them, enable communication and coordinate activities, create a platform for coordination. However, the mandate here is not strong enough to impose anything. It is up to the Member States to take specific actions. The situation is different in the field of food safety, where EU institutions such as EFSA have a much stronger mandate at the EU level. In the field of public health, however, this is not the case, there are only soft legal instruments that can be used, therefore a crucial role is played by the coordination and support of the Member States in their activities.

JO: How did the cooperation between the European Center for Disease Prevention and Control and the Member States look like?

PK: It was happening on many levels since the beginning of the pandemic. We are used to such contacts. Compared to the US's CDC, or even to national public health institutes, we have less than 300 people on the job — which is not so much, therefore, we constantly collaborate and rely on collaboration with outside experts. This is, of course, our bread and butter. There are several mechanisms that we have launched very quickly in a pandemic: one is the ECDC Advisory Forum, which normally meets several times a year to advise ECDC on priorities, what we should work on, how, and how they see issues from their perspective. It is a body made up of major national epidemiologists, mostly heads of public health institutes and experts in infectious disease epidemiology. Of course, when the pandemic started, Forum meetings focused on COVID-19. We often met online to discuss the situation, share information, and listen to what they had to say. One of the main instruments used to communicate during a pandemic was called the rapid risk assessment. These are documents that describe the situation at a given moment, as well as predictions and options for measures that countries could take concerning that situation. Then, from this "menu", countries can choose the measures that suit them best. Of course, the situations vary greatly from country to country. We have prepared approximately a dozen rapid risk assessments last year and we always consult with the member states through the Advisory Forum. On the other hand, when we cooperate with experts in thematic fields, we always include all Member States. We have a network of experts called ECOVID — they discuss details, especially about epidemiological surveillance, or, to put it differently, case definitions. From the beginning of the pandemic, we have made efforts to standardize how data should be collected. There are also a lot of topics, related to laboratory work, on the methods of coronavirus detection. For example, when the rapid antigen tests were starting to be used, we were working closely with our network. This is our permanent working method. Even before the pandemic, we had a dozen or so expert networks in the main fields, such as HIV/AIDS, tuberculosis, and vaccine-preventable diseases. Now we have created an additional ECOVID network. At the technical and expert level, we have good contacts with them, meetings are organized every week. We also cooperate with the World Health Organization — especially with the European office in Copenhagen. In the field of vaccines, we also have a virtual platform, called NITAG Collaboration (National Immunisation Technical Advisory Committees), where we have representatives from each Member State. They are representatives of advisory committees advising Member States' health ministries on vaccination programs. Therefore, we have an online platform where specialists share their plans, about which groups and whom they will vaccinate. Therefore, from the very beginning, there was very intensive cooperation with the Member States. Initially, it took the form of more cooperation on epidemiological surveillance, collecting data, control options, however, over time the focus has shifted to vaccines. Even if there is no strong legal mandate from the European Union in this regard, such cooperation is very beneficial. Of course, in the end, each of the Member States makes their own decisions — that is why there are so many differences between countries when it comes to restrictions placed on their territory.

JO: What was the cooperation and coordination of activities with the WHO like?

PK: From the beginning of the ECDC's existence, we have been cooperating with the World Health Organization. The office of the European region is located in Copenhagen, where our experts contact and coordinate our actions at least once a week. We inform them about what we are working on, what recommendations we plan to issue, we try to coordinate it with what the WHO is doing. It is difficult at times because they have a different field of action. The European office of WHO covers fifty countries, reaching the region of the Pacific — once the USSR belonged to this office, after the collapse of the former Soviet Union, former bloc countries remained in the area of operation of the European office, i.e. the countries of the Caucasus and Central Asia. There is quite a diversity of systems and economic situations there. So sometimes the recommendations issued by the European office of the WHO have to be adapted to very different situations. We have to issue recommendations that target the European Union, where the economic situation and technological advancement are often different. So there are discrepancies and discussions. One thing we had to work out at the start of the pandemic was the definition of cases —so that there would be a single, uniform definition. It was important in order for us to know how the data is collected and how we decide upon the number of cases of COVID, to make sure that we are talking about the same thing. Our cooperation with the WHO's global office in Geneva is based on the fact that we participate in the large webinars they organize to know what is planned at the global level. The natural partner, however, is the European office.

JO: How did the cooperation with non-European agencies and research centers go, and what were the examples of this cooperation?

PK: We have signed the memoranda of understanding with several epidemiological centers around the world. In the previous year, we organized, from time to time, online meetings of those centers that happened to have the time to meet and we talked about the situation in our countries and continents, shared what we were planning, and exchanged experiences. In addition, there were bilateral contacts regularly when needed. One such situation occurred in early April last year, when we radically changed our approach to the use of masks outside the health sector, by the general population. Based on previous data, that is, studies that were conducted mainly in the field of flu prevention, it appeared that face masks were not effective in protecting people from infections on the street or in people who do not work in the healthcare sector. They were generally reserved and recommended in the health service. At the beginning of April, however, data began to appear that they are also effective for people outside the health service, i.e. in everyday situations. We coordinated this quite closely with our colleagues from the CDC in Atlanta, the United States because they had fairly early studies in their area that proved the effectiveness of the masks. They considered changing attitudes and recommending the wearing of masks by people outside the health service. We coordinated our actions with them and at the beginning of April, we issued recommendations, which were a big change of approach on our part. Until today, when I give interviews, people keep asking questions about it. This is perhaps due to a misunderstanding of how science works. I get questions about why we suddenly changed our mind: „before you said the masks didn't work and now you say they work," for example. That's just how science works, especially medical science — as information is gathered, new evidence emerges that may at some point change an established paradigm, and we change recommendations. Coordination with colleagues from other centers often helps here, to avoid situations where there are divergent recommendations because it undermines some confidence in public health.

JO: What, from your perspective, were the biggest challenges for the ECDC during the pandemic? What can you be proud of?

PK: As I mentioned before, the duration of this pandemic is certainly a challenge that required organizational adjustments in our center. At some point, with a longer crisis, not everything can be dealt with by crisis response mechanisms, as there are projects that will be long-term, such as work on vaccines. We had to organize it organizationally in our normal structure, that is, remove it from the field of crisis response. This happened in September last year. We also had to adapt to the situation on an ongoing basis, due to the duration of the pandemic. The success is undoubtedly the reception of what we produce, as we received feedback that our guidelines are often used in formulating national recommendations. Although we do not have a legal basis to impose anything on European law, many Member States follow the recommendations we suggest. This kind of feedback motivates our employees a lot. After all, it is hard work, often on weekends and above standard working hours. But you have to keep working because the pandemic does not stop.

JO: How can we view the future of health policy in the European Union? What are the plans for the ECDC and the entire organization?

PK: There is a European Health Union project at the European level and the health program has received much more funds. It is very positive, a lot of things are happening here. However, in the context of our agency, we have received a lot more funding for 2021 — especially for research related to vaccines and especially for their effectiveness in widespread use outside of clinical trials. Vaccines are no longer used in clinical randomized trials, but in very large trials in everyday life. Very large funds are needed for this, so we got extra money, as well as some extra jobs. We are currently recruiting. So there is a reaction to what is happening. Hopefully, this will stimulate a global increase in healthcare spending and more investment in vaccine and drug research and become something like a wake-up call as to what is important when it comes to financing and investing in medicine and research.

JO: What was your role in the production of vaccinations and implementation of vaccination programs? Did you follow the test results on an ongoing basis during the testing phase?

PK.: We work very closely with the European Medicines Agency, but the registration process itself — that is, the very process of scientific evaluation of clinical trials and other information — is their domain. This process was slightly modified during the pandemic because the Medicines Agency introduced the so-called rolling review, i.e. a continuous process of analyzing the clinical data that fell to them. This meant that when a phase of the study was completed, the company could submit the results to the European Medicines Agency without waiting for the final application. This made the registration process a lot faster. At that time, we analyzed the data that emerged and we worked very hard with the advisory bodies advising ministries and governments in the Member States to build vaccination programs. In every European country and most countries around the world, there are committees of experts who are officially nominated to design and suggest what a country's immunization program should look like. Aside from the pandemic, historically, first, of course, came the childhood immunization programs, but currently, vaccinations are increasingly moving towards , life long' or ‚life course' programs, as adults are vaccinated more and more often. At some point last year, these committees began to prepare plans in the event of authorized COVID-19 vaccines: Who will we vaccinate, which age groups, which groups of the population, how, will it be normal channels, will there be special campaigns and special vaccination centers? These advisory bodies are called NITAGs, or National Immunization Technical Advisory Groups, we also have an online platform called NITAGs collaboration platform. We created it before the pandemic because it is badly needed. It provides an opportunity for collaboration and coordination of national research into vaccination programs. Vaccination programs are completely uncoordinated, as countries differ in who they vaccinate, have different epidemiological situations, structures of health care, and often even education, which affects vaccination. The platform, however, helps coordinate vaccine research, and we have used it when COVID-19 emerged. Since the middle of last year, this platform (NITAGs collaboration platform) has had meetings often every week, for example, comparing who we will be vaccinating in neighboring countries. It was learning from each other using data, as one needed to build a strategy based on data, which at the beginning was scarce. Hence, it had been said and it is still the case, that vaccination programs are flexible, they are open, they are not fixed once and for all and as we obtain more data, they will be adapted. This collaboration was very intense and resulted in the publication of a document on vaccination strategies in the EU last year. For our part, we have a mathematical modeling team that wrote a document based on mathematical models showing what populations to vaccinate and what the effect will be. This is a document from December 2020, which is available on our website. It says that in the beginning, it will be most effective to vaccinate the elderly and those with comorbidities as there will be too few vaccinations. It also confirms that vaccination of younger people in the first line will not be a priority, as there is no good data yet that vaccines slow down the transmission of the coronavirus. We only know that they protect against disease. We could do a lot, even though the data was very incomplete. However, our role is increasing right now, because when the European Medicines Agency suggests authorization to the commission, vaccines enter a large market and this gives an opportunity for extensive research on their

effects in clinical practice (what we call the real-life studies). We are starting a project in this area with the European Medicines Agency — which will
monitor safety, while the ECDC will monitor vaccine effectiveness.

JO: What are the groups of problems that should be considered during a
pandemic? How does the recommendation to the Member States look like?

PK: There are many groups of problems. One concerns the so-called non-
pharmaceutical interventions. In Poland, it is called restrictions, but it's a
negative word. We call them ‚non-pharmaceutical interventions'. At the beginning of a pandemic, there are no medications — this is where the use
of masks, physical distancing, and handwashing come into play. It sounds
trivial, but there are a lot of problems behind it. When someone starts to go
into it, we start getting very detailed questions. If you look at our website,
there are detailed documents on topics such as: How much time should you
wash your hands? It is not enough for a person to rinse them — one needs
to find data on the effective length, for example, the basis for the recommendation that it must be at least 20 seconds. What to disinfect your hands
with? What is the physical distance to be? The WHO suggests 1.5m, we say
2m, US CDC 6ft. It's not that after two meters this virus is gone, and up to
two meters there is, but you have to find a middle ground somewhere. We
also say that if someone is at least 15 minutes within 2 meters of an infected person, the chance of infection is very high. So as we start delving into
this, more and more factors come into play. However, we need to issue some
guidelines, we cannot just stay at the stage of summarizing the scientific data
and, for example, tell people that this is a continuum and that the probability of infection decreases with distance. This is one important group of such
recommendations. Another issue concerns masks: what types of masks are,
in what situations to use them, how to disinfect them. Masks, especially the
more advanced ones with the FFP2 mask filter, can to a certain extent be dis-
infected and used again. We also had to look into this. So there are a lot of
problems here. Later, once we publish such guidelines, we are getting some
more specific questions. When we published our case diagnosis guidelines,
there were questions about what to do when a person has a positive PCR
test three months after having a disease. In the beginning, there were recommendations that such a person must be in the hospital, but you cannot
keep someone in the hospital for 3 months. Now many countries do not let
such people in — they cannot travel because they have a positive test all the
time. The question is how to tell if a person is still contagious or not. There

are ways to do this, so we get specific questions and we have to answer them. Our microbiologists have to decide upon some recommendations. These are further examples of the complexity of many topics and the need to find practical recommendations for tackling the pandemic. Recently, new variants of the virus have been a hot topic, which is why we are talking to the WHO about the so-called variant assessment framework to evaluate which variant is worrying and which is not. There are many of these variants, the virus has mutated quite significantly because as an RNA virus it mutates at a certain constant rate. The longer it is with us, the more variants will appear. We have to ask ourselves which variant can create problems for us and we have to monitor it. It turned out that the Member States sequenced a very small percentage of virus isolates. We are not talking about PCR detection, to detect new variants, you have to sequence the genome, that is, determine the exact sequence of nucleotides. Here, many countries sequence less than 1% of the isolates, so we can be said to be essentially „blind". We are making a great effort in this direction to allocate funds to help countries sequence as many percent of isolates as possible. So there are some examples where we need to really go deeper and work with countries to help them align what they do. One area in which it is relatively difficult for us to unify something is what is happening at national borders. We try to scientifically provide the basis for recommendations on what to do, who to test, who to quarantine when traveling and crossing borders. However, it is difficult because it includes non-scientific arguments, various political arguments, reciprocity, and many more. So we try to scientifically provide some basis so that countries can make decisions based on our recommendations — of course, taking into account their own circumstances and conditions. We published some more information on this in the last risk assessment from January 2021. Here, there was a change because before there were disturbing signals about the so-called „variants of concern", we said that border blocking is rather ineffective in terms of inhibiting transmission, including border testing and post-arrival quarantine. We suggested that if resources were limited, it was better to use them to combat epidemics at home and in the population than to spend them at borders. Now we have changed the perspective as new variants are often more transmissive, often 50% easier to become infected with. In the last risk assessment, we are giving more recommendations as to what to do at the borders, for example, we encourage to limit the so-called non-essential travel.

JO: When it comes to the issues of *borders* and lockdowns, there were also problems with supply chains.

PK: Yes, here the European Commission reacted very quickly and created the so-called "green lanes". I do not know if it broke through to the media, but it took a lot of work to enable the flow of goods —especially medical supplies, used in the health sector, so that despite the closed borders not block transport and allow inter-landings of planes. Here, the European Commission has worked very hard with the Member States to allow the flow of key goods. We are also talking about the movement of people, for example, health workers, who travel, and these restrictions should not be applied to them. It seems that this is often a natural reaction to close borders in the face of danger, but it carries with it dangers.

JO: You mentioned the insufficient sequencing of isolates — these are problems that appear over time. Were there any other anomalies that you as the ECDC noticed as the pandemic unfolded?

PK: The whole sphere of laboratory testing is very important. It's always the case at the beginning of a pandemic that there aren't many laboratories that can test and detect a new pathogen. Here, we are working with a laboratory network that helped countries that did not have the capacity to test at first. Samples could be sent to laboratories that already could diagnose COVID-19. We worked very intensively with them in the initial period of the pandemic. If a country did not have the ability to detect the virus at all and there were few infected people, it could send samples to a laboratory that is on our network. In the beginning, there were two such laboratories — in Berlin and the Netherlands. At the beginning of the pandemic, it was possible to send samples there. Then, of course, all countries began to be able to test the cases at home, but there were also problems with the number of samples that could be tested. There was a shortage of reagents and laboratory equipment. When the pandemic hit us in full in March 2020, there was a period of exponential growth in infections and there were plenty of samples to be tested. This is often the case with large epidemics, therefore in this area, there was a lot of cooperation. At one point, we also had to help the European Commission by preparing the algorithm for Remdesivir distribution— this is an antiviral drug that works in certain situations. Admittedly, there has been controversy with clinical trials, but there are indications that in some patients with severe COVID, this drug may help and shorten hospitalization. So there was a problem with the division of doses, the number of which was limited. Of course, we help the European Commission all the time on the epidemiological side. There are still open questions, such as the question of schools and the role of children in the epidemic. In this regard, COVID-19 is different from the flu - with the latter, schools and children play a big role in transmission. In the case of COVID-19, it is known that children become infected and can infect others, but we have not seen schools becoming the seedbed of an epidemic. In our guidelines, we have tried to find some kind of middle ground so that the schools would work, but would operate safely. School closure for very long periods has very negative non-medical consequences. Of course, the Member States themselves make their own decisions in this regard, but we have produced documents for them on this subject to help them make these decisions. In general, we say that closing schools is the last resort — when the transmission volume cannot be reduced by other means.

JO: What were the controversies with Remdesivir?

PK: Remdesivir has been studied in large clinical trials where the results were published at different times. Based on the early results, the picture was more optimistic. Agencies such as the European Medicines Agency and the US FDA began recommending the use of Remdesivir. Then they limited it when new study results emerged, especially from the large WHO clinical trial called "Solidarity". However, this is how it works in medical science that as new results come in, dosing patterns or target groups are often limited or changed. The situation is developing and you need to respond to it. However, in some media, it sounded as if it were some kind of mistake because the recommendations had to be changed. This is how science works, it is a continuum— today we know less, tomorrow we can know more and we have to adapt.

JO: Disinformation in the media must be a nuisance when working in such an agency.

PK: Yes. We try to maintain the closest possible contacts with the media. You can have the best guidelines, but if they are not properly communicated then what we see now is happening, the so-called "pandemic fatigue", fatigue with all these restrictions. So we try to work with the media and deliver our message to reach the widest possible group of people. We try to show the light at the end of the tunnel and present some bright sides of the situation. This is important and the media can help us a lot. We have very live-ly contacts, we get a lot of inquiries asking for interviews and we try to use this to provide our guidelines and also encourage people to visit our website, to read more. We have a lot of infographics and videos on the website, with instructions on, for example, how to put the mask on correctly and how to wear it. I noticed that it is very often said that you just have to wear a mask — and then when a person goes out on the street and sees these masks being worn, he sees a different reality. We began to realize that it is not enough to say that you have to put on a mask, you have to show exactly how to do it. This is just one small example of how important the media is, it is often an amplifier of what we do and communicate.

JO: Have the coronavirus pandemic and the failure of health systems increased the risk of other diseases?

PK: Certainly. Our mandate is limited to infectious diseases, so we cannot really deal with chronic diseases, but the impact is certainly there. We can see it in research in the field of chronic disease prevention or cancer diagnostics. If wards are clogged, emergency rooms, emergency departments treat large numbers of patients with COVID-19 and suspected COVID-19, all diseases must be affected. What we are seeing from our perspective is the effect of vaccination. In some countries, during the initial period of the pandemic, childhood vaccinations were suspended — because there was a desire to reduce the flow of people through medical practices and the opportunity to become infected with COVID-19. This will certainly affect the diseases that we prevent with vaccines. We will grapple with the consequences for years, not only in COVID-19 but also in other diseases. However, there are also positive aspects. On the one hand, of course, it is difficult to talk about the positives when there is so much suffering, but the level of investment in health care changes. mRNA vaccines or vector vaccines are relatively new technologies. It is promising that, with the next new pathogens, it will be possible to create vaccines very quickly based on these innovative technologies. These platforms are likely to be used against existing pathogens such as influenza as well. Some of these mRNA vaccines have been designed to prevent Zika virus infection and other diseases. There is a lot of progress and I hope this trend will continue. Everything we are learning to combat COVID-19 will likely pay off in the next pandemics. We can see that drugs that work against COVID-19 also work against the flu. We currently do not register seasonal flu at all. Our surveillance system, surveillance, works, and samples are collected, but we hardly register the flu there, and usually, in

February it is already. The same was observed in the southern hemisphere when it was winter there, there was hardly any flu epidemic. So probably these agents are very effective also against other diseases that are transmitted by airborne droplets.

JO: What is the European Union's action in the field of health when it comes to helping the countries of the global south and neighboring countries? Is something like that happening and are these countries turning to ECDC?

PK: Yes, there are no borders in the field of health. Viruses do not respect borders, so we have to cooperate very much with centers from other continents. Whatever happens in Africa or Asia is immediately in Europe. When there was an Ebola epidemic in West Africa, we sent our experts there to help and fight on the spot. On the one hand, it is a matter of solidarity, on the other hand, by helping them, we are also helping Europe. Now the situation has slightly changed because for some time there has been a new agency, Africa CDC, with which we have contact and a joint program of very close cooperation. During the pandemic, we have weekly teleconferences as part of the Africa Task Force during which the situation in Africa is discussed. The cooperation is very close, also with the countries of the so-called "EU neighborhood", covered by the so-called "neighborhood policy" of the European Union. This applies, for example, to cooperation with the countries of the southern neighborhood, with the countries of the Mediterranean basin. We work here as part of the MediPIET (Mediterranean Program for Intervention Epidemiology Training). EPIET (European Program for Intervention Epidemiology Training) is our training program for epidemiologists, called field epidemiology. You can apply for it and, after qualification, take part in a two-year program, where you are assigned to a training center in the European Union. We have modular training that we do during these two years, plus you work in a good center and teach practical epidemiology. The first branch of such a program for the countries of the Mediterranean Basin. Collaborating with others is important. This is a necessity, there is no public health epidemiology without global action.

JO: As long as everyone is not healthy, nobody will be healthy.

PK: Yes, that's right.

Interview with Stephen Nagy, February 19th 2021

Dr Stephen R. Nagy is a Senior Associate Professor at the Department of Politics and International Studies at International Christian University in Tokyo. He is a Distinguished Fellow at the Asia Pacific Foundation (APF) in Canada, a Fellow at the Canadian Global Affairs Institute, and a Visiting Fellow at the Japan Institute for International Affairs (JIIA). He obtained his PhD from Waseda University in International Relations in 2009 and worked at the Department of Japanese Studies at the Chinese University of Hong Kong as an Assistant Professor from December 2009 to January 2014.

Beata Bochorodycz (BB): How COVID-19 has influenced Japan's position in the regional and global systems (supply chains, alliances)? Has any of Japan's foreign relations changed fundamentally because of COVID-19?

Stephen Nagy (SN): COVID-19 has not transformed but accelerated the process of selective decoupling from the Chinese market. From the Japanese government standpoint, they already have had problems with the supply chains and political unreliability of bilateral relations with China, and I think the first concerns about that came when Koizumi (Jun'ichirō) was a prime minister. He was visiting Yasukuni shrine and there was an informal boycott of Japanese products and then in 2010 when Chinese fishermen were arrested for colliding with a Coast Guard vessel, there were the rare earth embargos and then following the 2012 nationalization of the Senkaku islands under the Noda administration, we saw months and months of anti-Japanese demonstrations that caused damage to Japanese businesses in the eastern coast of China. So, I think these all have been critical junctures and Japan already has been thinking about how to recalibrate its economic and trading portfolio with China, and as result, many businesses were already moving to Southeast Asia and South Asia, not decoupling from China but the idea was China Plus One, and One was ASEAN countries.

And the Japanese government as early as 2010 already started to diversify certain supply chains, such as the rare earth materials supply chain. And they started looking to Mongolia, Myanmar, Tajikistan, Southcentral Asian states that have rare earth materials. And the labour cost has been pushing Japan to rethink its position in China. But China has amazing advantages in terms of speed, in terms of size, of the seasonal workforce and that comparative advantage it's not easily changed.

But the covid-19 period shocked the Chinese system, and the China-based global production system. And this affected Japanese businesses. In fact, it affected all the businesses. The Japanese government made a conscious decision to act more proactively, started to selectively recalibrate their relationship with China. There are some examples of that. In early May and late April, the Ministry of Finance passed a supplementary budget, which had two important parts. One was to provide some funding for reshoring of Japanese businesses to Japan and another part had a statement about strengthening the resilience and diversifying global supply chains. This budget allocation was important for starting the process of selective decoupling. And then in September 2020 the Indians and the Australians together with the Japanese signed an agreement called Resilience Supply Chain Initiative. This initiative is meant to diversify supply chains through Southeast Asia and South Asia.

If there is another big shock to the Chinese system these other supply chains can take over, so it will not impact the Japanese economy much. The third level of this is driven by geopolitics, the rivalry between Japan and China, but more broadly between the United States and China. The Trump Administration has already started putting pressure in 2018 with the trade war, putting tariffs on anything that was made in China. And of course, this affected Japanese businesses in China as well. That was another driver that has been pushing Japanese business to find a better balance between the Chinese market and Southeast Asia and South Asia market. And I think the Trump Administration also put a lot of pressure on Tech supply chains and the Tech supply chains are even more important in terms of semiconductor companies and limiting semiconductor companies' ability to manufacture and get parts that can be used in Chinese technological supply chains.

These are all drivers that have been shifting Japan's thinking about its relationship with China and its relationship with Southeast Asia and South Asia.

If you talk to policymakers here in Japan the general view is that we cannot divorce ourselves from China, we need the big Market, the supply chains there, and the production networks are irreplaceable today. But at the same time, we need to move forward with the concepts like Free and Open Indo-Pacific vision. We need to embed ourselves into the broader Indo-pacific region through economic partnerships, through partnerships that focus on Resilience Supply Chains Initiative, through trade partnerships so that Japan is firmly embedded into Indo-Pacific regions' broader economy. And that is to balance China.

BB: Which decisions of Japan's government during the pandemic do you consider (most) consequential for Japan's position in the international system?

SN: There are a couple of areas that you may want to look into. In October 2020 Japan hosted the Quadrilateral Security Dialogue (QUAD) between India, Japan, United States and Australia and I think that was significant. The leaders came together despite the pandemic to discuss and further institutionalize the quadrilateral security dialogue. And what was interesting about that when you read the discussions, there was less of a focus on China and more of a focus on trade and economy and supply chains diversification. So, I think that's important in further institutionalizing a new institution that is going to deal with the Indo-Pacific region that lacks a lot of institutions.

Second, you may think this is unrelated to the pandemic, but we did have the visit of Scott Morrison from Australia, and they signed a commitment to a defence treaty between Australia and Japan. What significant about this is that it has what is called reciprocal basing rights, so Japan can go and train in Australia and vice versa. Scott Morrison will come back next year and finalize it once they have dealt with the death penalty issue. And I think that demonstrates that Japan is becoming more... I don't want to say independent of the United States, but it's diversifying its security strategy, so it has the United States alliance as one pillar but also deepening strategic partnership with countries like Australia. And I expect that we will see more of these kinds of relationships over the coming years.

Third, I think it's also important for us to be thinking about how Japan dealt with pandemic domestically. Both South Korea and Japan did something marvellous. They didn't shut down the whole countries and violate all the human rights of citizens to get control of the virus. In both places, the deaths are relatively low and the infectious are relatively low. So, I think that it's important that they demonstrated a counterexample to the Chinese model that the central governments or authoritarian rule is the most effective way to deal with these kinds of issues. And I think that story needs to be written about much more as that the democracies (are capable of dealing with it as well). Of course, the United States is a disaster, but Australia, New Zealand, South Korea, Taiwan, and Japan have done relatively well compared to other countries. So, I think they have demonstrated that their systems are relatively effective in dealing with these kinds of issues.

I would also add that Japan continues to demonstrate leadership in pushing the Regional Comprehensive Economic Partnership (RCEP) forward. So, they signed the RCEP in November. What's important about this is that it demonstrated that Japan doesn't have a zero-sum approach towards China, neither does Australia or other members. And I think it's important to send the message to Washington that the countries in this region although they have many problems with China, they don't want the zero-sum approach to China. And again, Japan was one of the key players in pushing the original comprehensive economic partnership forward, and importantly in returning ASEAN back to the centre of East Asian regionalism or East Asian regional integration. I think when you compare it to BRI, BRI is really a China-centered form of integration from east to west, and the Free and Open Indo-Pacific model or vision that Japan is proposing puts ASEAN at the centre of regional integration, of growing supply chain diversification, of economic trade agreements as well. These are all quite important.

Last, Japan worked with Canada and Singapore and few other countries to try relaxing sanctions against some countries in Southeast Asia so they can get personal protective equipment. And again, this demonstrates pragmatic flexibility when and how we should enforce sanctions. Japan is not particularly wedded to human rights overseas and that allows it to have a little bit more flexibility and be less dogmatic in this area.

BB: Do you think that QUAD could begin the institutionalization process of FOIP?

SN: I think that QUAD is moving forward, especially QUAD Plus. QUAD, the four members will do more of the heavy lifting on the maritime domain in terms of maritime domain awareness, trying to keep the sea lanes of communication open. But the QUAD Plus is various forms of multilateralism and various forms of the corporation. For example, Canada is interested in the QUAD, but what can Canada bring? Most of it is capabilities that it can bring, like humanitarian assistance and disaster relief, good governance, some infrastructure connectivity in terms of skills. When we look at QUAD Plus, the substance of the activities would be very broad. In this sense, it could fit under the FOIP vision. Because FOIP vision has at its core peace and stability which is based on infrastructure connectivity, development promoting rule-based order, particularly in the maritime domain. They have really moved away from the strict securitization of the FOIP. An article FOIP 2.0 by Professor Hosoya Yuichi in the *Asia-Pacific Review* is very informative. I think the QUAD is going to continue to evolve into those countries that are front-lining or forward-leaning in terms of pushing back against China and the other countries that are really going to focus on development issues, infrastructure connectivity, diversification of supply chains, and likely some kind of health cooperation.

BB: What do you think about the timing of the Japan-Australia defence pact? Just after signing the RCEP.

SN: In September 2020, Japan signed Resilience Supply Chain Initiative with India and Australia, and then they held Quadrilateral Security Dialog in October, then Scott Morrison visited Japan, then they signed the RCEP. We see that Japan is engaging with China and trying to join organizations that will incorporate china into more rule-based organizations. So RCEP it's not high rules like TPP but it is still important. Japan is trying to engage China and at the same time hedging against China through these defence partnerships and multilateral partnerships. This is something that Japan continues to do even with regards to China joining the TPP. When Xi Jinping said that we can positively consider it (joining TPP), the Japanese said well, the standards are really, really high and the countries that meet the standards can join. That is not saying that you cannot join, China, but in reality, it is just like saying you cannot join. We continue to see this hedging process: engaging in China, trying to socialize China, trying to shape it from within, at the same time hedging significantly through strengthening the US-Japan alliance and creating other strategic partnerships, as we saw it with Australia. India-Japan partnership is very solid, Vietnam-Japan, The Philippines-Japan, as well. The Japanese have been courting the French the British, the Canadians, the Dutch to get a better view of the region.

BB: How do you evaluate Japan's domestic countermeasures for fighting the pandemic?

SN: This is tough. I think there have been problems with messaging when the ship *Diamond Princess* arrived at Yokohama Harbor in February. There was a problem with messaging there both with the domestic part of messaging and the international part of messaging. The Japanese public and international community found Japan's approach to the *Diamond Princess* to be poor, but again when you compare it to other cruise ships that were stuck in Australia, Hong Kong, and New York, the Japanese approach looked pretty humane and pretty good. This is how you tell the story.

Prime minister Abe without consultation with experts stopped schools in March last year, which, I think without proper consultations, doesn't make sense. It didn't allow for proper preparations for families to take care of their children to be able to manage to have children at home. These are shortcomings but these are shortcomings related to the fact that it was a novel experience. We didn't understand the severity of infectiousness of covid-19. It was a burden for many families. I talked to Taniguchi (Tomohiko) the former special adviser to prime minister Abe, who said flatly that the Japanese government was not prepared for students to study at home, to do everything online at home. Universities on the whole had to struggle. International Christian University was one of the first universities to go fully online in April. But even prominent national universities didn't come online until May. These are definitely some shortcomings, the messaging, and explaining what is happening.

After the first state of emergency, we saw the numbers dropped quite significantly but some people were still critical. And the numbers again spiked up in December and January but now they are dropping. The fact that they dropped so significantly over six weeks is a positive indication of government policy. And like most governments, they are struggling with how to deal with the businesses that are closing down, how to deal with the drop in consumption. Japan has been comfortable with financial socialism, always willing to give money out. It's always a question of balance, whether to get it out as quickly as possible or to have a more targeted approach and give it to the people that need it. As a policymaker, you have to make that decision. Probably five years from now people will look at the Japanese response and say it was maybe B minus. Because the number of deaths was low, the number of infections was low compared to other countries, even compared to Korea by proportion. But the economic impact was hard. It really showed the weaknesses of corporate Japan in terms of not being able to adapt to telework very easily. Many of the schools were doing stuff by paper and they couldn't adapt quickly to the demands of online education which is ultimately the responsibility of the government. Successive governments failed to prepare the country for the 21st century. And I think there is criticism about how they responded to foreign residents, who initially were not allowed to come back. Now they're treated the same as Japanese. You get a COVID-19 test and then do a quarantine.

I think they have a mixed record. Some of it is structural, some is cultural, some of it is related to the fact that it was a novel issue that's nobody knew how to deal with.

ABOUT AUTHORS

Piotr Baranowski - a fourth-year PhD candidate in political science at the Faulty of Political Science and Journalism of Adam Mickiewicz University in Poznań. In 2016 he defended his M.A. thesis Cybernetic-based State Power Measurement and in 2017 he began working on his PhD thesis entitled Meta-systemic Transformation Model. Complexity Paradigm. The author is interested both in the theory of International Relations and politics of the Arab World, during his PhD education he visited the Middle East multiple times (Iran 2017, University of Jordan 2019, University of Sulaimaniyah, Iraq 2019–2020).

Beata Bochorodycz – an associate professor (prof. UAM dr hab.) at the Institute of Oriental Studies of Adam Mickiewicz University (AMU) in Poznan. She holds MA (Japanese studies) from AMU and MA (political science) from Kyushu University in Japan, PhD and habilitated PhD (dr hab.) from the Institute of Political Studies of the Polish Academy of Science in Warsaw. Recipient of scholarships from the International Rotary Club, Japanese Ministry of Education, Japan Foundation, and Fulbright Foundation. Work and research visits at the Graduate School of Law Department of Kyushu University, Yokohama National University, Sigur Center for Asian Studies at George Washington University in Washington D.C., School of Oriental and African Studies (SOAS) in London, and National Graduate Institute for Policy Studies (GRIPS). Her research focuses on diplomacy and foreign policy of Japan, the US-Japan relations and Okinawa issue, decision making process in public administration, civil society, social movements.

Radoslaw Fiedler – a Professor at Adam Mickiewicz University (AMU), Poznan in Poland, head of Doctoral School of Social Sciences at AMU and head of the Department for Non-European Political Studies at the Faculty of Political Science and Journalism. Chairman of the Fiedler's Foundation. He is also the initiator and chairman of the international conference: Beyond Europe. The author of numerous articles and monographs on the Middle East and related issues, especially on the policies of the European Union and the United States of America. He is also the recipient of many grants and scholarships. He has given lectures at: Tehran University, Jordan University, Tianjin Technology University in China, Qaboos Sultan University in Oman, Cairo University in Egypt, Al Farabi National Kazakh University in Kazakhstan, Grigol Robakidze University in Georgia, Jakarta University in Indonesia, National Chengchi University in Taiwan. In the academic year 2019–2020, Fiedler was a visiting scholar (the Bekker Program – the Polish National Agency for Academic Exchange) at the Arnold A. Saltzman Institute of War and Peace Studies.

Rafał Kamprowski - Assistant professor at the Department of Security and Defense at the Faculty of Political Science and Journalism at the University of Adam Mickiewicz in Poznań. A graduate of MA studies in the field of history - he graduated with the Dean's award of the Faculty of History (2009), supplementary studies in the field of political science (2012). In addition, he completed postgraduate studies in internal and international security at the Faculty of Political Sciences and Journalism of Adam Mickiewicz University in Poznań (2015). He is the author of scientific articles and monographs in the areas of safety in environmental threats, food security, raw material safety, rare earth elements.

Jarosław Kardaś – an assistant professor at the Department of Non-European Political Studies at the Faculty of Political Science and Journalism of the University of Adam Mickiewicz in Poznań (AMU). PhD in the field of politics and administration. Participant of many conferences and author of several scientific publications on the processes taking place in the former USSR area. Lecturer in the field of security and international relations in the region of the South and North Caucasus and crisis management

Julia Orłowska – a student of international relations at Adam Mickiewicz University in Poznań. Her research interests focus on genocide studies, human rights, and contemporary threats and conflicts. In addition to her academic work, she co-founded and leads the educational project "Globalna Wioska".

Przemysław Osiewicz –an associate professor at Adam Mickiewicz University in Poznan, Poland. FULBRIGHT Senior Award Visiting Scholar at Walsh School of Foreign Service, Georgetown University, Washington D.C. (2016–17). Non-Resident Scholar, the Middle East Institute, Washington D.C. (2017-). A member of the Polish Accreditation Committee (2020–2023). A co-organizer, with Prof. Radoslaw Fiedler, of an annual international conference Beyond Europe. Visiting lecturer of universities in the United States, Cyprus, Belgium, Sweden, Pakistan, Turkey, Iran, and Taiwan. Author and co-author of five monographs and over 100 book chapters and articles in political science and international relations.

Sang-Chul Park – Professor. He has received PhD degrees in political science in Aug. 1993 in Germany and economics in Feb. 1997 in Sweden. His dissertations discussed Technopolises in Japan. He also passed a habilitation examination (full professorship) in political science in Nov. 2002 in Germany as well as a docent evaluation (Swedish habilitation) in economics in Sep. 2004 in Sweden. A Full Professor at Graduate School of Knowledge based Technology and Energy, Korea Polytechnic University. He was an Adjunct Professor at Center for Science-based Entrepreneurship, Korea Advanced Institute of Science and Technology (KAIST), and a Visiting Professor at Seoul National University, South Korea. He was also a Private Dozent at Justus Liebig University in Giessen, Germany and Visiting Full Professor at Gothenburg University, Sweden. He served as Associate Professor at Gothenburg University, Sweden from 2001 to 2003 and as Associate Professor at Okayama University, Japan from 2003 to 2006. He also stayed as Visiting Professor at Fudan University, China in Sep. 2014 and as Visiting Scholar at Asian Development Bank Institute, Japan in Oct. 2014. His research interests concern industrial policy and regional development and studies on innovation systems and on science parks and innovative clusters in particular. Currently his research areas are expanded toward energy policy, sustainable development strategy, high technology ventures and international business and trade.

Zuzanna Pawłowska - a student of international relations at the Faculty of Political Science and Journalism at Adam Mickiewicz University in Poznań, majoring in the world economy and international business. Her research interests focus mainly on human rights abuses, discrimination against minorities in the world, social and economic policies with an emphasis on mental health promotion, and culture and politics of SouthAmerican countries. In addition to her academic work, she is co-founder of the „Globalna Wioska" initiative.

Artur Pohl – an assistant professor at the Department of Non-European Political Studies at the Faculty of Political Science and Journalism of the University of Adam Mickiewicz in Poznań (AMU). He received the PhD in social sciences in the field of political science with a specialization in security policy in 2016, defending the dissertation entitled The main determinants of Israel's security policy at the beginning of the 21st century. Participant of many international and national scientific conferences, author of numerous publications and member of the Polish Society of Political Sciences.

Jakub Rösler – a student of international relations at the Faculty of Political Science and Journalism at the Adam Mickiewicz University in Poznań, majoring in diplomacy and consular relations. Research interests focus on the Middle East, Unrecognized States, in particular Transnistria. In addition to his scientific activities, he co-founded and runs the educational project "Globalna Wioska".

Maria Spychała-Kij – a third-year undergraduate in International Relations and Arab Studies at Adam Mickiewicz University in Poznań. She is interested in the field of international conflicts and humanitarian crises as well as the theories of IR. Former intern at the Centre for International Peace and Stability in Islamabad, exchange participant at Bilgi University in Turkey, author of a couple of papers published in peer-reviewed journals.

Rafał Wiśniewski – an assistant professor at the Strategic Studies Department, Faculty of Political Science and Journalism, Adam Mickiewicz University, Poznan, Poland; his research interests include: international security of the Indo-Pacific, great power competition and military strategy.